T0150257

PAIN RELIEF
through
TRADITIONAL CHINESE MEDICINE

Massage, Gua Sha, Cupping, Food Therapy, and More

By Liu Naigang

SCPG

Text by Liu Naigang
Translation by Shelly Bryant
Design by Wang Wei

Editor: Cao Yue

ISBN: 978-1-93836-884-4

Address any comments about *Pain Relief through Traditional Chinese Medicine* to:

SCPG
401 Broadway, Ste.1000
New York, NY 10013
USA

or

Shanghai Press and Publishing Development Co., Ltd.
Floor 5, 390 Fuzhou Road, Shanghai, China (200001)
Email: sppdbook@163.com

Printed in China by Shanghai Donnelley Printing Co., Ltd.

1   3   5   7   9   10   8   6   4   2

Contents

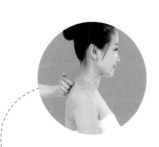
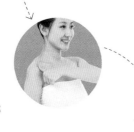

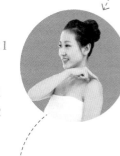

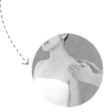

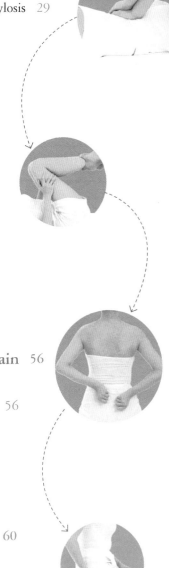

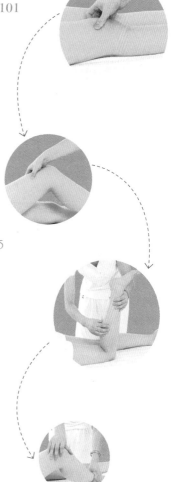

Preface

Pain in your neck, shoulders, back, legs, knees ... Are you
suffering from these issues? Chronic pain can be very detrimental
to a person's health. These conditions may seem mild, but they
will eventually develop into potential health hazards if not
treated. When the pain becomes severe, you will find it to be
a serious problem. Bad habits should be corrected early, at any
time in our daily life, before these seemingly small problems
develop into more serious issues that go beyond our control and
begin to affect our quality of life.

This book explains the various symptoms of neck, shoulder,
lower back, leg, and knee pain. It offers solutions such as
massage, scraping, moxibustion, cupping, exercise, food therapy,
and other traditional Chinese medicine (TCM) physiotherapy
methods to correspond to the various symptoms. If you follow
the methods suggested, based on the symptoms of your problem,
there will be an obvious improvement.

Treatment for neck, shoulder, lower back, leg and knee
pain is a long-term process. Follow the methods in this book
persistently, and you will keep these pains at bay. Early action is
also early prevention.

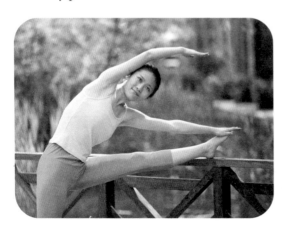

Doing exercise to
relax the body.

Chapter One
Identifying the Causes of Pain

Today, 70% of people suffer from chronic neck, shoulder, lower back, and leg problems. Bad habits and long periods of time in a fixed position can be the cause of these ailments. These small and seemingly harmless problems that occur intermittently are often ignored. However, they can actually be hidden chronic diseases. If they are not attended to and corrected, they will cause even more suffering.

People with neck, shoulder, lower back, and leg pains share similar occupational characteristics. For example, editors, programmers, and drivers have a very high probability of having such ailments. Most of these people have the same work characteristics, such as working in a sitting position or bending over at a desk for prolonged periods of time, excessive use of air conditioning and fans in summer, significantly decreased outdoor activities and physical exercise, high tension at work, as well as less sleep. Many people in this group suffer from neck problem and herniated discs.

Many people sit at a computer desk all day. Long-term bad posture, including bending over to read or write, stiffens the neck, increasing cervical pressure, muscle fatigue and tension, and leading to vertebral artery distortion, resulting in cervical spondylosis or cervical muscle strain. Another harmful work-related position is an improper lumbar posture. This causes a weight overload to the spine, rupturing the fibrous ring of the lumbar intervertebral disc, resulting in lumbar disc herniation and compressing the root of the nerve. This is why urban people today still suffer from neck, shoulder, lower back, and leg pain even with excellent working and living conditions.

1. What Is Chronic Pain?

Toothache is not a disease. People who have experienced it understand this, but it still causes agony. Toothache is only one sort of pain. You may also encounter problems such as lower back pain, leg pain, and shoulder pain.

It is easy to understand why the medical community calls pain the "fifth vital sign" after breathing, the pulse, body temperature, and blood pressure. There are two types of pain, namely acute and chronic. Acute pain is only a symptom of certain diseases. It comes and goes quickly. When you catch a cold, you may get a headache. In its most serious state, the headache becomes very intense. When the cold is gone, the headache will also disappear. It does not linger for long.

Chronic pain, on the other hand, can last for a while, ranging from a month to several years. Such pain is slow and faint, and becomes intense on rainy days or after over-exertion. Acute pain is easier to treat than chronic. Once the illness is cured, the pain will disappear. Chronic pain treatment is more cumbersome. Although some of these pains will not affect normal life, they are bothersome nonetheless, and reduce the quality of life.

2. Bodily Pain

Neck. The principle of human biomechanics states that the human spine is an S-shaped structure composed of four physiological curves: the neck, chest, lower back, and sacrum. The cervical and lumbar vertebrae protrude forward, while the thoracic and sacral vertebrae deflect backward. This is to increase the elasticity of the spine, reduce harm to the human body from gravity, and protect the spinal cord and brain. If your head is always down, its center of gravity will incline forward. The cervical spine will also bend forward, and its lordotic curve will gradually disappear, or even protrude backward. Medical research has found that the disappearance and abnormality of this cervical curve are among the most common causes of cervical lesions.

Moreover, if the head is always leaning forward, the muscles and ligaments at the back of the neck will be in a continuous state of tension and fatigue, and the muscles of the neck will begin to strain. Statistics show that every time a computer is put into use, there will be two more neck pain patients. Although we cannot choose our working environment, we can protect our cervical spine. Bad habits such as spending too long surfing the Internet, playing computer games, and watching TV should also be avoided as much as possible.

Shoulders. The shoulder is a ball-and-socket joint that is very flexible. It can bend, stretch, retract, extend, rotate, and move in circular motions. There are many muscles around the shoulder joint, and they play a significant role in maintaining its stability. However, there are lesser muscles below the anterior joints, and with the joint capsule being very loose, the stability of the joint is therefore very poor. Improper posture for people who work with computers all year round is very likely to cause shoulder pain. People who do housework over a long period of time or people who overuse their shoulder joints often have pain in this area as well.

Back. Bending down to lift objects will likely lead to lower back pain. When picking up heavy things from the ground, we usually bend our body but keep our knees straight. Although this posture requires less effort, it basically depends on the back muscles. Therefore, these muscles and ligaments bear a huge burden, and become a risk factor for injury to the lumbosacral muscles and ligaments. If this continues for a long period of time, pain will surface in the weaker muscles and ligaments of the lower back.

Legs. The reason people are able to move flexibly and freely is due to muscle movements, and these excitations and contractions are the work of calcium ions. When blood calcium increases, it inhibits the excitability of muscles and nerves, and helps muscles relax. When the blood calcium is lower than 70 mmol/L, the excitability of neuro-muscles will increase, and the skeletal muscles will experience pain and convulsions. A considerable element of leg pain and muscle cramps that many middle-aged and elderly people experience is caused by a calcium deficiency.

Calcium is the most plentiful mineral in the human body. About 99.3% of it is concentrated in the bones and teeth. Calcium plays a very important role in the metabolism and health of the human skeleton. However, the hormone levels in the body will decrease gradually with age, and bones will slowly lose their calcium. Thinning will begin to occur in the bone cortex, and the trabeculae will be sparse, atrophic, soft, and fragile. The medical term for this pathological change is osteoporosis. People in middle or old age are more prone to calcium deficiency. This is because the human body's absorption of calcium reduces significantly with age while the loss of calcium worsens.

Knees. Exercise is a good thing, but doing it incorrectly can cause aches and pains, such as sore knees. The knee joint is the most vulnerable part of the human body. This is because it has little protection in the form of fat or muscle. Movements such as running, squatting, and jumping need good knee function. Knee pain caused by inappropriate exercise is becoming a common phenomenon. This is especially so for the elderly, as the knee joint is prone to the effects of aging. Any inappropriate movement is likely to lead to injury.

3. Identifying Incorrect Posture

Habits like sitting still for a long period of time, resting your head on the table for a nap, crossing your legs, and reading in bed may be very comfortable in the moment. However, such positions subject the body to an abnormal curvature, and soreness will eventually surface. The following are types of incorrect posture:

Sitting in a sedentary state. Sitting for a long period of time without moving will increase the compression of the lumbar intervertebral discs. Riding or driving on poorly maintained roads causes the body to jolt and shake, and if there is a sudden braking of the vehicle, there is a risk of cervical joint dislocation. In turn, this will affect the corresponding nerves, causing neck and shoulder issues, or back and leg pain. Serious cases can result in cervical and lumbar disease.

Crossing one's legs. When maintaining the correct sitting posture, the sagittal plane of the human spine is an S-shape curvature, that is, the cervical vertebrae and lumbar vertebrae are forward convex, while the thoracic vertebrae and sacral vertebrae are backward convex. People tend to slouch when they cross their legs. If this continues for a long period of time, the normal physiological curve of the spine will be damaged, leading to issues such as lower back pain, muscle strain, and varicose veins. The habit of leg-crossing should be stopped early.

Slanted standing posture. Many people tend to stand askew. Once formed, this habit may tighten or loosen the left, right, front, and rear low back muscles that were originally symmetrical and coordinated. They will lose balance, causing uneven stress to the ligaments, fascia, and small joint capsule. Health issues such as hunchback, lumbar curvature, and pelvic displacement can easily develop.

Resting your head on the table. After waking up from a nap on the table, the most obvious feelings are a stiff neck, numb and weak arms. If the symptoms are severe enough to affect your daily work, you should take serious note, as it may cause cervical spondylosis. Poor posture from resting your head on the table can cause nerve compression, and in serious cases, possible hand paralysis.

Frequently wearing high heels. Spending a lot of time in high heels is detrimental to the spine. It increases the lumbosacral angle, and raises the chances of developing lumbar spondylolisthesis. It also increases the chances of lumbar intervertebral joint dislocation, and irritates the lumbar nerve, causing lower back and leg pain. In addition, wearing high heels regularly can cause the arch of the foot to gradually collapse, leading to flat feet. When this happens, the weight-bearing function of the foot will weaken.

Reading in bed. When we lie in bed and read a book, the neck will be flexed forward, which will cause the posterior longitudinal ligament, the ligamenta flava, the interspinous ligament and the ligamentum nuchae of the cervical spine to be in a state of tension, and cause excessive muscle tension in the relevant muscle groups. At this time, the inferior vertebral articulation at the top slides into the upper part of the superior vertebral articulation at the bottom, resulting in a misalignment of the joint surfaces and tension in the joint capsule. At the same time, the intervertebral disc, which should be relaxed and recovered by lying on its back, is squeezed at the front because of the forward flexion of the neck, the nucleus pulposus moves backward, and the posterior fibrous ring is strained. In the long run, it will lead to soft-tissue damage, which will accelerate the degeneration of the vertebrae, intervertebral discs, and surrounding soft tissues. Eventually, cervical spine problems will occur due to pressure on the spinal cord, nerve roots, and vertebral arteries.

Incorrect bending. Incorrect bending will cause lower back pain. When bending forward, the external force on the lumbar spine is greater, especially the lumbosacral force. If your knee is not bent and you bend quickly, the stress on the lumbar joint will increase, which can easily increase the pressure on the lumbar intervertebral disc, causing a sudden sprain, and resulting in symptoms such as lower back pain.

Cold lower back. The lower back is the part of the body that is most vulnerable to cold. If it gets cold, it will cause contractions of the small blood vessels and muscle spasms, increasing the likelihood of intervertebral disc herniation. Moreover, the lower back corresponds to the kidney in TCM. One of the functions of the kidney-*yang* (refer to page 118) is to warm the whole body, while the normal function of the body is maintained by *yang qi*. Once cold sets in to the lower back, the kidney-*yang* will be damaged. Because the kidney-*yang* governs the bones, the lumbar spine will also be affected.

Taking a nap in a moving vehicle. This is bad for your spine. Any sudden acceleration or deceleration of the vehicle jolts the body forward and then back, causing a lot of damage to the cervical spine. If you feel that your cervical spine or lumbar spine have been injured during a ride, you must not try to fix it yourself. There are a lot of nerves in the spine. You may incur further injuries with improper movement, risking paralysis. The best thing to do is to go to a hospital immediately.

4. The Roots of Chronic Pain

Neck, shoulder, lower back, and leg pain are becoming increasingly common. These conditions seem to indicate a problem in a certain part of the body, but in fact, the root is in the spine.

The spine is the most powerful bone pillar in the human body. It is connected to the skull at the top and the tailbone at the bottom. It is composed of five parts: the cervical spine, thoracic spine, lumbar spine, sacral bone, and tailbone. It plays a very important role in normal life and activities, protecting the brain, spinal cord, and internal organs by supporting the body's weight and reducing the impact of shocks. The spine also enables us to perform actions such as forward flexion, backward extension, lateral flexion, and rotation.

The spine undertakes a major task, and its work is onerous and complex, making it vulnerable to fatigue. More importantly, as the body's most important nerve tissue, the spinal cord is distributed in the tube formed by the spinal vertebrae vertically from top to bottom. Why is the spinal cord so important?

Most of the nerve tissues on the body's surface and in the internal organs extend from the ganglion of the cervical, thoracic, and lumbar spinal cord, and are then distributed in the limbs and body. That is to say, all of the nerves of the skin and internal organs originate from the spinal cord. Therefore, if something goes wrong with the spine, it can affect all parts of the body.

These important functions of the spine, coupled with its susceptibility to fatigue and injury, naturally make it a high-risk area for various forms of chronic pain. The majority of the cases of neck, shoulder, lower back, and leg pain are related to it.

Bodily pain is often a sign of spinal disease. At present, more than a hundred diseases have been found to be related to the spine, including some that people would never have thought of, such as arrhythmia, headaches, vertigo, stomach pain, diarrhea, high blood pressure, and sexual dysfunction.

Diseases caused by the spine can involve the human nervous, respiratory, digestive, urinary, and endocrine systems. They can involve departments such as internal medicine, surgery, neurology, endocrinology, gynecology, pediatrics, otolaryngology, ophthalmology, and even dermatology. Many of the sub-health symptoms of modern times are caused by misalignments of the spine.

5. Checking Your Spine

How to find out if your spine is healthy?

When standing, both shoulders should be on the same horizontal line. The spine should be straight, perpendicular to the ground, like a pine tree. When sitting, the lower back should be straight, with the torso tilting slightly forward, the thighs and calves making a 90° angle, and the weight of the body resting stably on the pelvis like a bell drum.

If you experience any of the following issues, you may have a problem with your spine:

• The heels on the soles of your shoes often wear out unevenly. The cause of this problem is usually a difference in leg length, or uneven pressure exerted on the long axis of the spine.

• Taking full deep breaths has become difficult.

• Your neck, back, or joints on other parts of body make a cracking sound, which is usually caused by joint dysfunction in the small joints of the spine.

- Your head or hips are not able to twist or rotate easily to the same angle on both sides, and your range of motion is gradually reduced.
- You often tire easily. An unbalanced spine drains your energy.
- Concentration becomes difficult, as spinal discomfort affects the brain.
- You are susceptible to disease and illness. Spinal strain and other issues affect the normal immunity of the neuroendocrine system.
- Your feet point outward when walking. This could be a sign of problems in your lower spine or hips, or uneven pressure in your head, neck, and base of the skull.
- Your standing posture is incorrect. Proper posture consists of standing with your feet apart at shoulder width, with your body weight equally distributed on the soles of both feet. Otherwise, the spine, head, or buttocks are not on the center line of the body.
- You get headaches, and pain in your neck, lower back, back, and muscles or soft tissues of joints. These are usually signs of spinal strain or other lesions.
- Your back and neck feel stiff and uncomfortable. This is also a sign of strain or other spinal lesions.

6. Caring for Your Spine

As the pillar and nerve center of the human body, the spine is directly or indirectly related to many problems and conditions. Therefore, you should make an effort to safeguard your spinal health and avoid issues. Smoking is strictly discouraged, and alcohol should be limited. Exercise and physical work should be carried out daily. Combine work and rest, and maintain an optimistic and happy temperament to avoid excessive mental tension. Taking care of your spine when you are young will slow down the aging process.

A simple way to maintain spinal health is through massage

therapy. The spinal nerves connect the brain to the rest of the body, and these nerves pass through the intervertebral foramen of the spine. Massage therapy can have a great relaxing effect. However, if the massage methods and techniques are wrong, it can be hazardous to spinal health. For example, too much pressure during massage therapy can lead to edema, tension, and muscle stiffness. More seriously, long-term repeated deep pressure massage on the spine can damage its stability, accelerate the degeneration of the intervertebral discs, and cause severe stress to the spinal cord. Moreover, massage therapy is not suitable for some spinal lesions.

In traditional Chinese medicine, the kidneys govern the bones, and are related to the growth and development of marrow and the function of the bones. The kidneys store essence[1], which produces bone marrow. When the bone marrow is plentiful, the bones are strong. The rise and fall of the essence and *qi* (refer to page 60) of the kidneys directly affect the growth, nutrition, and function of the bone structure. Therefore, to nourish the spine is to nourish the kidneys.

When there is sufficient essence in the kidneys, the bone density will be strong. The kidney essence is made up of two parts: one is the innate essence, which is directly inherited from our parents before we were born, and the other part is the acquired essence. The latter is built up after we were born, from the food nutrients transformed and transported by the spleen-stomach, and the nutrients metabolized from the various organ systems. The innate essence, which is the main component of the kidney essence, lays the base that is supplemented and nourished by some acquired essence. Therefore, the kidney *qi* transformed by the kidney essence is an innate *qi*.

Essence generates the production of marrow. The kidney

---

[1] Essence generally refers to the basic substances that constitute the human body and maintain life activities. It is divided into innate essence and acquired essence.

essence produces bone marrow, spinal marrow, and brain marrow. Bone marrow nourishes the bones. The kidneys store essence, which generates marrow production, and the marrow nourishes the bone. This constitutes a system that is internally related. There must be sufficient kidney essence to guarantee enough source material for the metaplasia of the bone marrow, which can then nourish the bones and increase their density and strength.

7. TCM Therapy to Relieve Pain

TCM physiotherapy is effective at alleviating and healing chronic pain if it is carried out consistently over a period of time. The following are the various methods of TCM physiotherapy.

Massage: also known as *tui na*—a form of traditional physiotherapy. After an injury, the muscle attachment points, tendons, ligaments, joint capsules, and other soft tissues produce traumatic and aseptic inflammatory reactions, sending out pain signals, and then causing reflex muscle spasm, which will aggravate pain. Massage can increase blood supply to the lesioned soft tissues, eliminate inflammation, reduce pain, and fully alleviate muscle spasm to relieve pain. It should be noted that most of the acupoints involved in the massage steps in this book are located symmetrically on the body. The diagram may show the acupoints on only one side of the body. Please refer to the description of the locations of these acupoints in the appendix. If they are symmetrical on both sides of the body, massage both sides. You can massage yourself, or ask someone to help with the places that you are not able to reach.

Moxibustion: using moxa as heat therapy, the application of a warm compress or herbal plaster on acupoints will produce warmth or chemical stimulation in the meridians. Moxibustion can then regulate *qi* and blood through the transmission of these meridians, which can strengthen the vital *qi* to eliminate pathogens[1], and enhance the body's ability to resist disease. Moxibustion is also able to remove blockages in the meridians through the heat it generates, as well as reducing swelling and removing blood stasis, eradicating toxins, and relieving pain. Through the effects of warmth and medicinal aromatic resuscitation, moxibustion can improve local blood circulation, relieve vasospasm and muscle spasm, and provide chronic pain relief.

Cupping: cupping is a technique in which negative pressure is created by applying a flame to a cup or pumping air out of it to create suction, so that it can be placed on the skin to form local blood stasis. Its therapeutic effects include dredging and vitalizing the meridians[2], dispelling pathogenic Wind and Cold[3], promoting the circulation of *qi* and blood, as well as improving detumescence and pain relief. To achieve the best possible results in the treatment and relief of pain, select the appropriate acupoints and persist for a period of time.

Gua Sha **scrapping:** scrapping or *gua sha* therapy stimulates the body's meridians and acupoints. It dredges and revitalizes the meridians and collaterals, promotes the wholeness of the meridians, and enhances the body's two-way regulation in strengthening resistance to eliminate pathogens. It is used to treat many conditions caused by excessive and deficient *qi* and blood, or chaotic *qi* movement in the meridians, and also

---

[1] Strengthening the vital *qi* to eliminate pathogens refers to a therapeutic principle in which *qi* is enhanced to improve the body's immune ability to dispel pathogenic factors that lead to illnesses.

[2] In TCM, a meridian is considered as a system that communicates between the exterior and interior of the human body and connects with the five *zang* and six *fu* organs inside the body. These meridians, which run vertically across the body, link the interior to the exterior and the top to the bottom of the body; the internal organs, extremities, and joints are responsible for carrying and distributing *qi* and blood to nourish the muscles and bones.

[3] Wind and Cold are both external causes of disease in TCM. Wind is related to the springtime, and is associated with the liver system. Cold is related to the winter and the kidney system.

enhances the functions of the various organ systems to which the meridians belong. *Gua sha* can also improve the human body's self-regulation, immunity, and rehabilitation in the treatment of local illnesses. It can strengthen resistance to pathogens, regulate *yin* and *yang*, invigorate health, and prevent and treat diseases.

In addition to the above, TCM offers physiotherapy methods such as herbal baths, herbal pillows (including for the lower back), and steaming to relieve pain. As these methods involve the use of many medicinal Chinese herbs that can be somewhat complicated, they are not mentioned in detail in this book.

Body Length Measurement

Using Thumb Length

The width of the patient's thumb joint is 1 cun. This is applicable for locating the acupoint on four limbs with vertical cun.

Using Middle-Finger Length

With the patient's middle sections of the bent middle finger as measurement, the distance between two inner crease tips is taken as 1 cun, which is mostly applicable for locating acupoints on four limbs with vertical cun and on the back with horizontal cun.

Using Four Fingers Closed Together

With the index finger, middle finger, ring finger, and small finger stretched straight and closed, measure at the level of the large knuckle (the second joint) of the middle finger. The width of the four fingers is 3 cun.

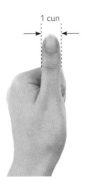

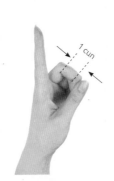

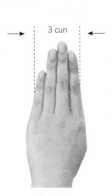

Chapter Two
Treatments to Relieve Neck Pain

Cervical spine problems no longer belong exclusively to the elderly, but are a problem that increasing numbers of young people are facing, especially those who work long hours in front of a computer. Sitting in the wrong position can lead to stiffness and muscle pains in the neck. If you remain immobile and do not move from time to time, this will slowly develop into chronic cervical disease over time, causing a great deal of discomfort. So, how can cervical vertebra diseases be prevented and treated? This chapter will explain.

1. Understanding Neck Pain

There are many signs of a bad cervical spine, such as sometimes feeling soreness in the head and neck, back of the shoulder, or arm, feeling stiffness in the neck, limited twisting activities of the neck, weakness in the lower limbs, and numbness in both feet. Do you have any of these symptoms? If so, it means that you may have a problem with your cervical spine.

Knowing about Your Cervical Spine
The cervical spine is the smallest of the vertebrae, but the most flexible, most frequently active, and heavily weighted segment.

The cervical spine is an important gateway through which nerves pass, both to carry instructions from the brain to all parts of the body and to transmit messages from the body back to the brain.

The cervical spine is the area located below the head and above the thoracic spine. The cervical spine is composed of seven cervical vertebrae. Except for the first and second cervical vertebra, there is an intervertebral disc between the other cervical vertebrae, plus the intervertebral disc between the seventh cervical vertebra and the first thoracic vertebra. There are six intervertebral discs in the cervical spine. Each cervical vertebra is composed of two parts: the vertebral body and the vertebral arch. The vertebral body is an oval-shaped column, and the vertebral body is connected to the vertebral arch, which together form the vertebral foramen. All the vertebral foramina are connected to form the spinal canal, in which the spinal cord is housed.

Reasons for Cervical Spine Problems

If you touch the back of the neck with your hand, you can feel a large bulge. Counting one segment up from here and six segments down, all of these belong to the cervical spine. Since humans began to walk upright, the load on the cervical vertebrae has increased significantly, because it carries a heavy head on its top.

The weight of an adult's head is around 4.5 to 5.5 kilograms. The slender cervical spine not only has to bear the weight of the head itself, but also a pair of sagging upper limbs hanging on both sides. The cervical spine is very mobile, with forward flexion, backward extension, lateral flexion, and rotation. It is this kind of pressure from the head and upper limbs over the years, as well as frequent neck activities, that makes the cervical bones, joints, and soft tissues very susceptible to injury and fatigue, thus posing a hidden risk of neck pain and dysfunction.

From the perspective of TCM, the cervical spine is located in the position of the Du Meridian (refer to page 77). This meridian starts from the perineum, follows the midline of the back spine upward, passes through the back of the neck, crosses the top of the head, and ends at the face. If the cervical spine is bad, there may also be problems with the Du Meridian.

Problems with the cervical spine cause soreness and pain in the head, neck, shoulders, back or arms, stiffness in the neck, weakness in the lower limbs, and numbness in the feet. What are the reasons for this?

• Looking at the computer or phone for a long time; sedentary behavior: keeping your head bent low for long periods of time will lead to stiffening of the neck muscles.

• Exposure to cold in summer: exposure to cold over prolonged periods with air conditioning turned very low.

• Late nights without sleep: insufficient sleep will cause the muscles to be in tensed condition, adding burden to the cervical spine.

Caution for Neck Massage

It should be noted that not every type of cervical spondylosis is suitable for massage. There are many types of cervical spine diseases, and their conditions are complex. Some may not be suitable for massage at all.

• Before deciding on a type of massage, check with a licensed hospital first. After getting a diagnosis based on your symptoms, you can then decide whether massage therapy is suitable and what kind of massage will best suit your problem.

• If you suffer from cervical spondylotic radiculopathy, massage can be done on normal days. However, when you get an acute attack, do not massage the neck. This may aggravate the inflammation and edema of the nerve root, and make the condition worse.

• People suffering from cervical spondylotic myelopathy should only receive gentle massage therapy. Strong stimulating massage and the method of pulling the cervical spine will not have a positive therapeutic effect, and may cause severe shock to the spinal cord leading to paraplegia.

2. Common Acupoints for Relieving Neck Pain

As one of the traditional methods of TCM treatment, massage can be effective for maintaining health, such as relieving spasm and tension in the neck muscles and ligaments, improving blood circulation in local tissue, restoring the normal structure of cervical vertebrae and joints, and inhibiting pain. It can also help with some neck conditions.

Most neck pain is caused by a lack of movement and prolonged incorrect posture that results in too much weight on the neck. When working or studying, it is best to turn your head every 45 minutes.

Six Main Acupoints

Fengfu point: to locate this point, follow the spine upwards to the skull, place one finger horizontally above the posterior hairline. The Fengfu point can alleviate headaches, neck pain and adverse activity caused by cervical spondylosis.

Tianzhu point: this point is located in the posterior area of neck, in the depression of the outer edge of the trapezius muscle. This point is the best choice for all kinds of headaches and neck discomfort.

Baihui point: to locate the point, sit upright. It is at the intersection of the tip of both ears and the midline of the head. Gently massage this point with your fingers every day to relieve dizziness caused by cervical spondylosis.

Fengchi point: this is an important point for eliminating pathogenic Wind, and is located below the occipital bone at the pool-like depression. People with cervical spondylosis who work at

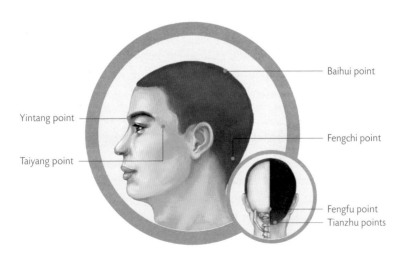

their desk for a long time should press the points with both thumbs.

Yintang point: this point is located at the midpoint of the line between the eyebrows. Daily massage can provide significant relief from headaches, dizziness, nausea, and other discomforts caused by cervical spondylosis.

Taiyang point: this point is located in the depression about one finger thickness away from the middle point connecting the tip of the eyebrow and the outer canthus. Kneading this point can alleviate ailments caused by cervical spondylosis such as headaches and vertigo.

Massage Tips

A variety of massage techniques can be used on the acupoints. You can massage with the tips of your thumbs, index fingers, or middle fingers, centering your movement around your wrist, shoulder, or elbow joint and knock with force on the affected area. Alternatively, you can press the acupoints with your fingers or palms, and apply downward pressure and stimulation to some parts of the body surface for certain time and with certain force, or use the pulp of your fingers to perform the pinching technique. This technique is sub-divided into 2-finger, 3-finger, and 5-finger pinches.

3. Massage Methods for Neck Pain

Besides cervical spondylosis, cervical pain is also caused by bad habits, incorrect posture, and other certain diseases. It can also cause discomfort to the other parts of the body. This section explains massage methods for different cervical spine diseases and for the various symptoms caused by cervical spondylosis.

Cervical Spondylosis

The symptoms of cervical spondylosis are pain and heaviness in the neck and shoulder muscle groups, and weakness in the upper limbs. This is often related to unsuitable pillows and bad sleeping posture. People suffering from this should use pillows that are of an appropriate height, and lie flat on their back in bed. They must exercise regularly, rest properly, and avoid being in a fixed position for long periods of time. They can also rub the back of their necks with their hands, combined with therapy methods like hot compresses, moxibustion, and cupping for pain relief.

Massage for 15 minutes once in the morning and once in the evening during an attack. During the recovery period, massage once a day for 15 minutes. For normal healthcare, massage 2 to 3 times a week, for 15 minutes each time.

Massage Points

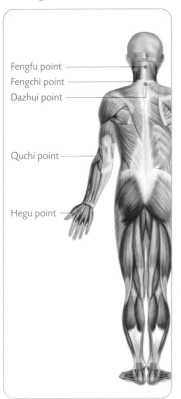

Fengfu point
Fengchi point
Dazhui point

Quchi point

Hegu point

Message Method

❶ The patient should be seated and relaxed. Stand behind the patient, and knead the muscles at the back of the neck from top to bottom with fingers repeatedly. Then, massage the Fengchi and Fengfu points on the neck, followed by the Hegu and Quchi points on the upper limb with the thumb. Ask the patient to gently turn their head and neck to the left and right.

❷ Place one hand on the patient's jaw and the other hand on the occipital bone at the back of their head. Tell the patient to relax their neck muscles.

Apply some force, lift, and pull slowly with both hands 2 to 3 times. The pressure should be adjusted for the patient. Avoid excessive force.

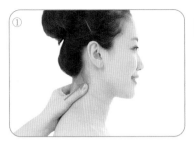

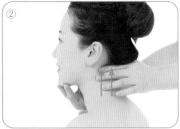

❸ Tap gently on both sides of the patient's neck and shoulders with two hands; at the same time, ask the patient to stretch, bend, and rotate their neck slowly and gently.

❹ Patient can bend cervical spine forward, and put four fingers of right hand together, place them on the highest ridge of the lower neck, and massage the Dazhui point by pushing and kneading repeatedly about 20 to 30 times, until the area feels hot.

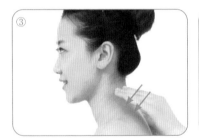

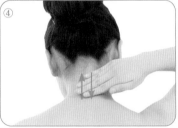

Cervical Spondylotic Radiculopathy (Pinched Nerve)

Patients feel significant neck pain and pressure in the paravertebral muscles, which is usually associated with irritation and compression of the spinal nerves. Patients should strengthen the muscles of the back of the neck and shoulders, relaxing the muscles and making sure not to compress the nerves. They can also rub the back of the cervical vertebrae with their hands and use methods such as *gua sha* scraping to relieve pain.

Patients can combine treatment with gentle massage.

Rough massage should be avoided. During an attack, massage therapy should be carried out once in the morning and once in the evening, with each session lasting 20 minutes. During the recovery period, massage once a day for 20 minutes. For normal daily healthcare, massage 2 to 3 times a week for 15 minutes each time.

Massage Points

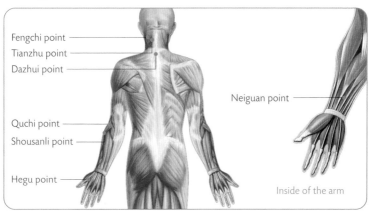

Fengchi point
Tianzhu point
Dazhui point

Neiguan point

Quchi point
Shousanli point

Hegu point

Inside of the arm

Massage Methods

❶ The patient should either be seated or prone, and relaxed. Use the pulp of fingers to knead the soft tissue along both sides of the cervical spine repeatedly, to relieve muscle spasms. Adjust the pressure according to the patient's tolerance.

❷ Use the pulp of fingers to knead and massage the tender area. Press and knead successively on the Fengchi, Tianzhu and Dazhui points.

For patients with arm pain and numbness, move from the upper arm to the forearm, press and massage the Quchi, Shousanli, Neiguan, and Hegu points.

❸ Support the patient's occipital bone with one hand and their lower jaw with the other hand, and gently turn their head several times.

❹ Patient can use the pulp of fingers and palms of both

hands to alternately tap the neck, shoulders, and arms, slowly moving the neck at the same time.

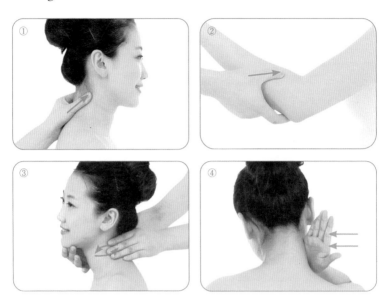

Vertebral Artery-Type Cervical Spondylosis

Dizziness, blurred vision, and memory loss are symptoms of vertebral artery-type cervical spondylosis, which is usually related to stimulation of the cervical vertebral artery. People suffering from this should correct their posture. They should not repeat mechanical movements for long periods, but balance work and rest, and avoid overwork. They should take time to rest, and eat more food that will boost the blood level in their diet. In addition to massage, methods such as cupping and moxibustion can be included to relieve pain.

During an attack, massage should be performed once in the morning and once in the evening, with each session lasting 30 minutes. During the recovery period, massage can be reduced to once a day for 20 minutes. For normal healthcare, 15 minutes of massage 2 to 3 times a week is sufficient.

Massage Points

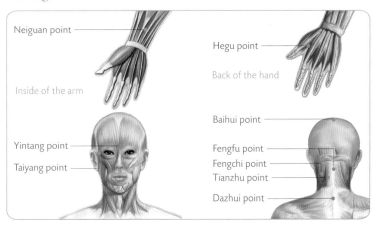

Neiguan point

Inside of the arm

Yintang point

Taiyang point

Hegu point

Back of the hand

Baihui point

Fengfu point

Fengchi point

Tianzhu point

Dazhui point

Massage Methods

❶ Put the patient in the prone position. Stand beside him/her, and knead and rub the muscles on both sides of the cervical spine, neck, and shoulders using the pulp of thumbs. Then, using the fingertips on both hands, apply pressure to the spinous process in the middle of the patient's cervical spine and the transverse process on both sides.

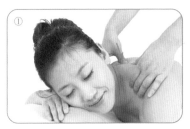

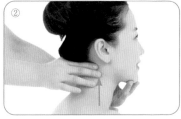

❷ Sit the patient up. With one hand, hold the occipital region of their head. With the other hand, hold their jaw. Gently lift and pull their neck up.

❸ Use the fingers of both hands to press the meridian points accordingly in turn: the Baihui, Yintang, and Taiyang points on the head; the Fengfu, Fengchi, Tianzhu, and Dazhui points on the neck; the Neiguan point on the arm; and the Hegu point on the back of the hand; massage each point for 2 to 3 minutes.

❹ Patient can place the pulp of four fingers onto the vertebral artery on both sides of the midline of the cervical spine, and gently rub from the neck and shoulder to the occipital bone.

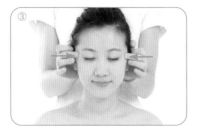
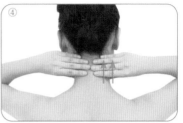

Sympathetic Cervical Spondylosis

This is related to intervertebral disc degeneration and segmental instability. People who suffer from this ailment should avoid over-exhaustion, and should not stay in a fixed position for a long time. They should drink plenty of water, stay calm, and take more bed rest.

During an attack, massage should be performed once in the morning and once in the evening for 20 minutes each time. During the recovery period, massage can be reduced to once a day for 20 minutes. For normal healthcare, 15 minutes of massage 2 to 3 times a week is sufficient.

Massage Points

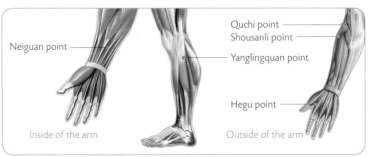

Neiguan point

Quchi point
Shousanli point
Yanglingquan point

Hegu point

Inside of the arm

Outside of the arm

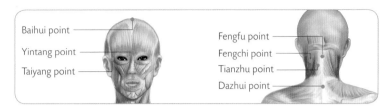

Baihui point

Yintang point

Taiyang point

Fengfu point

Fengchi point

Tianzhu point

Dazhui point

Massage Methods

❶ The patient should be seated and relaxed. Stand behind him/her and perform the rolling[1] and kneading techniques on their neck several times to relieve neck muscle spasm.

❷ Massage the meridian points of the head and neck, press the Baihui, Yintang, Taiyang, Fengfu, Fengchi, Tianzhu, and Dazhui points, followed by the Neiguan point in the arm and the Hegu point on the back of the hand. Apply gentle force, but do it repeatedly, so as to stimulate the points. When the patient is relaxed, get him/her to tilt their head backward slowly, extending the head and neck, then rotate their head from left to right several times.

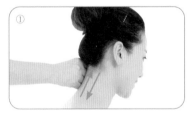

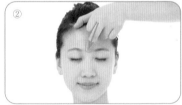

❸ Put the patient in the prone position. Stand behind him/her. Place one palm on the back of the other hand and gently press the cervical spine several times; avoid applying excessive force.

---

[1] Rolling technique: bend the fingers naturally, and lay the back of the fifth metacarpophalangeal joint on the acupoint. Relax your shoulder joint. Use your elbow joint as the pivot point, and use your forearm to drive the flexion movement of your wrist and the rotation of your forearm, so as to roll the back of your palm (with the third, fourth, and fifth metacarpophalangeal joints and the side of the hypothenar of the palm as the axis) back and forth continuously on the acupoint.

❹ Patient can use his/her thumb to press and knead the Quchi, Shousanli, Neiguan, Hegu, and Yanglingquan points on the opposite limbs alternately.

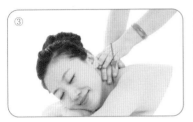

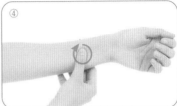

Headaches

The most common types of headache are vascular and neurotic. The causes of these ailments are usually related to vasodilation and contraction dysfunction of the head and dysfunction of the cerebral cortex. People who have these problems should avoid tiring their brain and becoming anxious and nervous. They should do frequent neck stretching exercises to relieve pain and relax the neck muscles. They should avoid over-exertion and get plenty of rest. Appropriate daily exercise coupled with *gua sha* scraping and moxibustion can help relieve headaches.

During an attack, massage should be performed once in the morning and once in the evening for 20 minutes each time. During the recovery period, massage can be reduced to once a day for 15 minutes. For normal healthcare, 15 minutes of massage 2 to 3 times a week is sufficient.

Massage Points

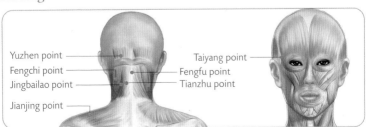

Massage Methods

❶ Patient can spread the fingers of both hands and hold the back of his/her head. Using both thumbs, one on each side of the Fengchi point, press and knead for 3 minutes.

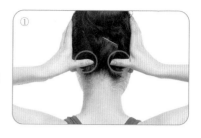

❷ Using the pulp of the thumb to press and knead the Fengfu point for 3 to 5 minutes.

❸ Place the pulp of the thumb on the Tianzhu point of the neck. Slowly press and knead, and gently apply pressure for 3 to 5 minutes each time.

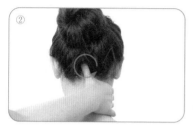 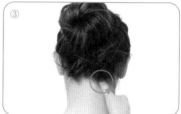

❹ Place the pulp of both thumbs on the Yuzhen points on each side of the head. Gently exert pressure, and slowly press and knead for 3 to 5 minutes each time.

❺ Close the gaps of the four fingers of each hand. Both hands perform the pinching technique with the thumbs on Jianjing points on the shoulders for 5 to 10 minutes.

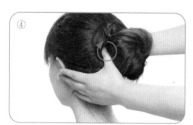 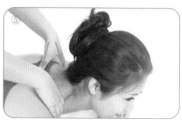

❻ Using the pulp of thumbs, gently press and knead the Taiyang points 30 to 50 times.

❼ Place the pulp of thumb on the Jingbailao point on the neck, and apply moderate pressure. Press the point 10 to 20 times.

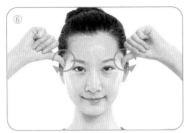

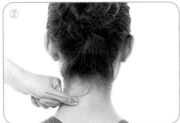

Stiff Neck

A stiff neck is often related to incorrect sleeping posture, inappropriate pillow height, or cervical spondylosis. People with this problem should change to suitable pillows, exercise regularly, and take proper rest. In addition, the hot compress method can be used to relieve pain. During an acute attack, immobilization is required.

During an attack, massage should be performed once in the morning and once in the evening, with each session lasting 20 minutes. When recovering, massage therapy can be reduced to once a day for 15 minutes each time. For normal healthcare, 2 to 3 times a week is sufficient, with each session lasting 10 minutes.

Massage Points

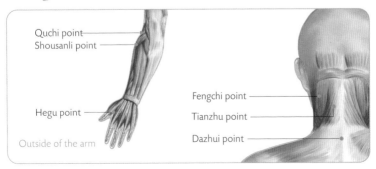

Quchi point
Shousanli point

Hegu point

Outside of the arm

Fengchi point
Tianzhu point
Dazhui point

Massage Methods

❶ The patient should be seated and relaxed. Stand behind him/her. Pinch and knead to relax the muscles on both sides of the neck and shoulders. Apply pressure from light to heavy, lasting for 3 to 5 minutes.

❷ Focus on pressing, kneading, and pinching the tender areas and the Fengchi, Tianzhu, and Dazhui points in the neck area. While massaging, let the patient carry out neck movements at the same time, such as forward flexion and back extension, right and left lateral flexion, and rotation.

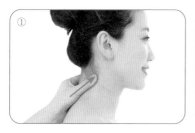
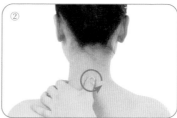

❸ Using the pulp of the thumb, press the patient's Shousanli point on the arm for several minutes.

❹ With both hands, the patient can alternately knead the Quchi and Hegu points on the opposite limb for several minutes, moving the neck at the same time.

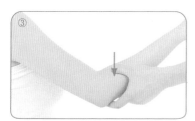
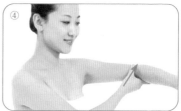

Numb Fingers

This is related to factors stimulated by hyperosteogeny arising from the degeneration of the cervical spine. During an attack, the fingers will not be painful nor itchy, but rather numb and uncomfortable. People with this health issue can apply massage and hot compress treatment on the acupoints on the neck and upper limbs. They can also perform some cervical stretching exercises, as well as relaxing their mind, taking proper rest, and not placing stress on the cervical nerve.

During an attack, massage should be performed once in the morning and once in the evening, with each session lasting 20 minutes. During the recovery period, massage once a day for 15 minutes. For normal healthcare, massage 2 to 3 times a week, for 10 minutes each time.

Massage Points

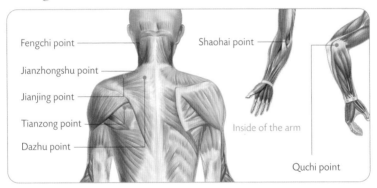

Fengchi point

Jianzhongshu point

Jianjing point

Tianzong point

Dazhu point

Shaohai point

Inside of the arm

Quchi point

Massage Methods

❶ Close the gaps between your four fingers, and together with your thumb, grasp and pinch the Jianzhongshu point on the patient's shoulder for 5 to 10 minutes.

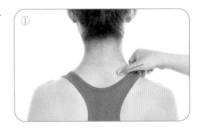

❷ Place both thumbs on the Fengchi points respectively, press and knead for 3 minutes.

❸ Close the gaps between your four fingers, and together with your thumbs, grasp and pinch the patient's Jianjing point for 5 to 10 minutes.

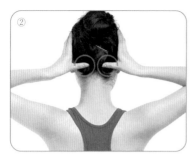

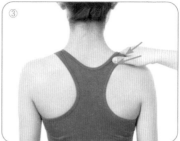

❹ Close the gaps between your four fingers, and together with your thumb, grasp and pinch the patient's Dazhu points on both sides of the shoulders for 5 to 10 minutes.

❺ Press and knead the Quchi point with the thumb for 3 to 5 minutes.

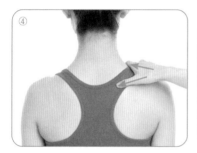

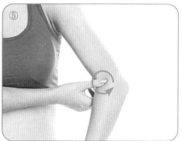

❻ Press the Tianzong point on the shoulder blade with the thumb 15 to 30 times.

❼ Press and knead the Shaohai point with the thumb for 3 to 5 minutes.

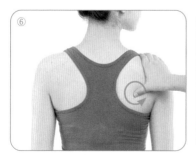

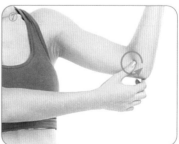

Palpitations

Palpitations manifests themselves through irregular heartbeat patterns that cause discomfort. This is due to the compression of blood vessels and nerve roots. If you suffer from palpitations, you should maintain a peaceful state of mind, get enough sleep, and consume proper nutrients. In addition, avoid strenuous exercise and excessive physical exertion over a prolonged period.

During an attack, massage should be performed once in the morning and once in the evening, with each session lasting 10 minutes. During the recovery period, massage once a day for 5 minutes. For normal healthcare, massage 2 to 3 times a week, for 5 minutes each time.

Massage Points

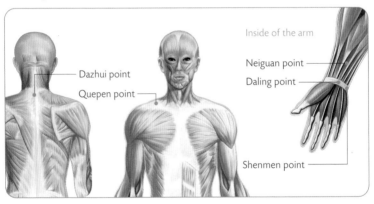

Massage Methods

❶ The patient sits up. Tilt his/her head slightly to the good side to reveal the shoulder and neck of the affected side. From the side of the neck to the top of the shoulder, perform the top-down rubbing and kneading. Repeat 10 to 20 times.

❷ The patient remains seated. Press his/her Dazhui point gently with the pulp of your thumb for 3 to 5 minutes, increasing the pressure until the patient feels a throbbing tenderness in the affected upper area.

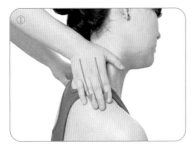

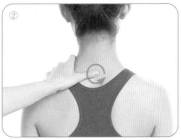

❸ Remain seated. Gently press and knead the Quepen point with the pulp of thumb for 3 to 5 minutes, increasing the pressure until there's a throbbing tenderness in the affected upper area. The exerted pressure should not be too intense to tolerate.

❹ The patient holds his/her wrist, with the thumb gripping the palmar side of the wrist and the four fingers holding the dorsal side. Pinch and knead the Daling, Shenmen and Neiguan points. Repeat this action 5 to 10 times.

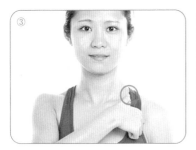

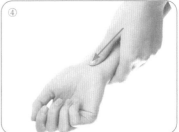

Vertigo

Vertigo is a spinning sensation of varying degrees, without an obvious shaking motion. It is usually related to the compression of the vertebral artery and excessive nervous tension due to cervical spine lesions. Sufferers should rest well and ensure adequate sleep, and undergo massage therapy often to reduce stress. In addition, maintaining a peaceful state of mind, keeping the surrounding environment clean and quiet, increasing outdoor exercise, and having therapeutic treatments such as moxibustion and cupping can help alleviate symptoms.

During an attack, massage should be performed once in the morning and once in the evening, with each session lasting 10 minutes. During the recovery period, massage once a day for 5 minutes. For normal healthcare, massage 3 times a week, for 5 minutes each time.

Massage Points

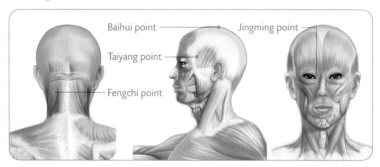

Massage Methods

❶ Gently press the Baihui point 30 to 50 times with the thumb.

❷ Gently press and knead the Taiyang points in circular motions with both thumbs 5 to 10 times.

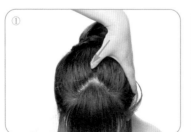
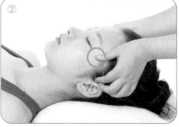

❸ Press the Jingming points with the pulp of thumbs or ring fingers, and knead in a circular motion 20 to 30 times, gradually increasing the pressure.

❹ Spread five fingers open. Hold the back of the head, place the thumbs on the Fengchi points on both sides, press and knead for 3 minutes.

❺ Cover both ears with the heel of both palms, and gently vibrate and press them rhythmically 2 to 5 times. Avoid using too much force.

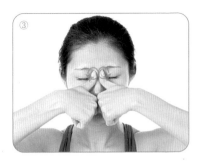

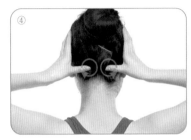

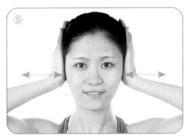

Deafness and Tinnitus

The symptoms are a ringing sound in the ear and varying degrees of hearing loss. These conditions are usually related to cervical sympathetic nerve dysfunction caused by cervical instability. Sufferers should get enough sleep, maintain a relaxed emotional state, and carry out self-care massage therapy to alleviate the condition. In addition, adequate rest, taking essential nutritional supplements, and avoiding strenuous exercise can also help.

During an attack, massage should be performed once in the morning and once in the evening, with each session lasting 20 minutes. During the recovery period, massage once a day for 10 minutes. For normal healthcare, massage 2 to 3 times a week, for 10 minutes each time.

Massage Methods

❶ Gently press and knead the Ermen point with the pulp of the middle finger for 3 to 5 minutes.

❷ Press and knead the Tinggong point with the pulp of the middle finger for 3 to 5 minutes.

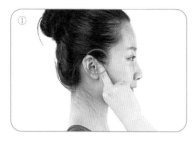
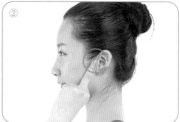

❸ Spread open the five fingers of both hands. Place the thumbs on the Yuzhen points on each side, and press and knead for 3 minutes.

❹ Press and knead the Tinghui point with the pulp of the middle finger for 3 to 5 minutes.

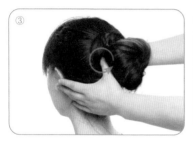
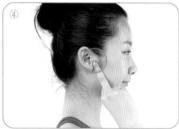

❺ Spread the five fingers open. Place the thumbs on the Fengchi points on both sides, and press and knead for 3 minutes.

❻ Press and knead the Yifeng point with the pulp of thumb for 3 to 5 minutes.

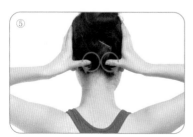
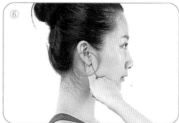

Massage Points

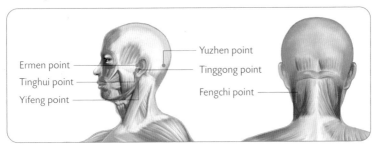

Ermen point
Tinghui point
Yifeng point

Yuzhen point
Tinggong point
Fengchi point

Lower Limb Weakness

The symptoms are feebleness, numbness, and heaviness when lifting the feet. In some patients, the pathological changes of cervical spondylosis are related to the spinal cord. Taking adequate nutritional supplements and getting enough sleep is vital. Carry out massage therapy to improve blood circulation in the thighs and lower legs. Try lying in bed to relax your body, and avoid strenuous exercise. In addition, other therapeutic methods such as moxibustion can help to alleviate symptoms.

During an attack, massage should be performed once in the morning and once in the evening, with each session lasting 10 minutes. During the recovery period, massage once a day for 5 minutes. For normal healthcare, massage 3 times a week, for 5 minutes each time.

Massage Points

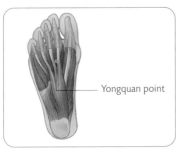

Yongquan point

Massage Methods

❶ Push-press the Yongquan point 200 to 300 times with the root of your palm, gradually increasing the pressure.

❷ The patient takes the prone position. Knock on and around the plump part of the patient's hips with hollow fist.

Repeat this action 20 to 50 times, either gently or with slight force.

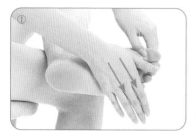
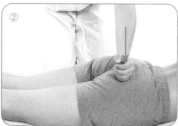

❸ The patient takes the prone position with lower limbs straightened naturally and knees slightly bent. Use both hands to perform the grasp-pinch-loosen technique around the patient's thighs and lower legs from top to bottom, and repeat 3 to 5 times.

❹ The patient takes the prone position, straightens the lower limbs naturally, and bends the knee slightly. Use palms to knead the inside and back of the patient's thighs, and the back and inside of the lower legs. Knead and move from top to bottom, and repeat 3 to 5 times.

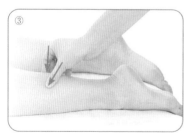
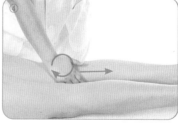

❺ The patient takes the supine position. Clench the fist and knock on the front and outside of the patient's thighs from top to bottom and from the inner to outer side, repeating this action for 5 to 10 times.

❻ The patient takes the prone position and lifts the soles of feet upward. Hold the patient's toes with one hand and punch the soles of feet with the other. The hammering has to be firm, steady, accurate and solid. Repeat this action 3 to 5 times.

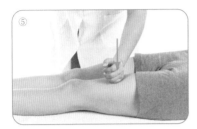
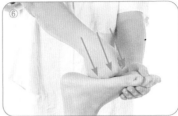

Tremors

Tremors are a rhythmic shaking of the body, usually related to cerebral ischemia caused by cervical spine lesions stimulating the sympathetic nerve and vertebral artery. Patients should maintain a peaceful state of mind and have enough sleep. They can relax local muscles through massage therapy. In addition, relaxing the body, keeping the air circulation in the environment obstruction free, and avoiding strenuous exercise can alleviate symptoms, coupled with physiotherapy like cupping.

During an attack, massage should be performed once in the morning and once in the evening, with each session lasting 20 minutes. During the recovery period, massage once a day for 10 minutes. For normal healthcare, massage 3 times a week, for 5 minutes each time.

Massage Points

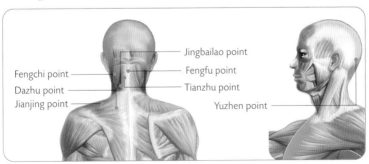

Fengchi point
Dazhu point
Jianjing point

Jingbailao point
Fengfu point
Tianzhu point

Yuzhen point

Massage Methods

❶ Spread open the five fingers and hold the back of the head. Place the thumbs on the Fengchi points on both sides of the head. Press and knead for 3 minutes.

❷ Press and knead the Fengfu point with the thumb for 3 to 5 minutes.

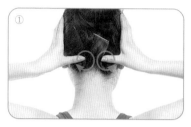
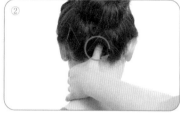

❸ Gently press and slowly knead the Tianzhu point on the neck with the thumb pulp for 3 to 5 minutes.

❹ Applying moderate pressure, press the Jingbailao points on the neck with the thumb pulp 10–20 times.

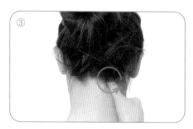
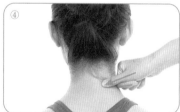

❺ Close the gaps of four fingers and together with the thumb, grasp and pinch the Dazhu point on each shoulder for 5 to10 minutes.

❻ Place the pulp of both thumbs on the Yuzhen points

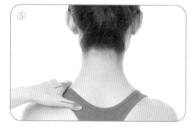

on both sides of the head respectively. With gentle force, slowly press and knead for 3 to 5 minutes.

❼ Close the gaps of the four fingers and together with the thumb, grasp and pinch the shoulder's Jianjing point for 5 to 10 minutes.

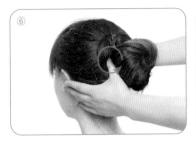
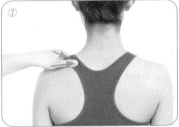

4. Other Methods for Neck Pain

Apart from acupoint massage, moxibustion, cupping, water therapy, exercise can also be used in combination to relieve neck pain. The heat generated from moxibustion can effectively relieve neck pain. Cupping can clear blockages in the neck and promote *qi* and blood flow. Water therapy can alleviate neck stiffness. Simple exercise for the neck can be done anytime, anywhere.

Moxibustion

When carrying out moxibustion therapy, it is important to note that the moxa stick should not touch the skin. Use suitable pillows. Proper rest should be allowed, as it is not good to remain in the same position for a long time. Moxibustion can be done once a day, but each session should not last too long. It should not be carried out of the patient who has a fever.

Moxibustion Points

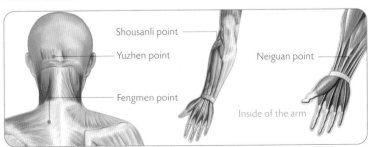

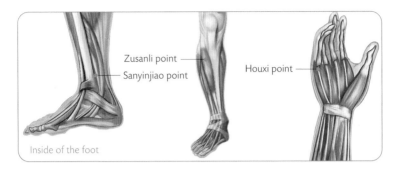

Zusanli point

Sanyinjiao point

Houxi point

Inside of the foot

Moxibustion Methods

❶ Ignite the moxa stick. Place it at about 1.5 to 3 cm away from the Yuzhen point, and hold it there for 3 to 5 minutes.

❷ Ignite the moxa stick. Place it at about 1 to 3 cm away from the Zusanli point, and hold it there for 3 to 5 minutes.

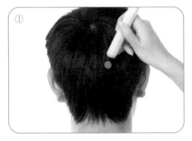

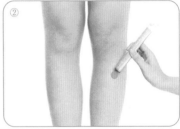

❸ Ignite the moxa stick. Place it at about 1.5 to 3 cm away from the Houxi point, and hold it there for 3 to 5 minutes.

❹ Ignite the moxa stick. Place it at about 1.5 to 3 cm away from the Fengmen point, and hold it there for 3 to 5 minutes. (Do not do it through clothes. The picture is only for illustration.)

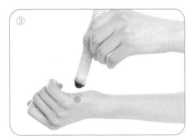

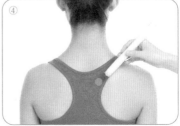

❺ Ignite the moxa stick. Place it at about 1.5 to 3 cm away from the Neiguan point, and hold it there for 3 to 5 minutes.

❻ Ignite the moxa stick. Place it at about 1.5 to 3 cm away from the Shousanli point, and hold it there for 3 to 5 minutes.

❼ Ignite the moxa stick. Place it at about 1.5 to 3 cm away from the Sanyinjiao point, and hold it there for 3 to 5 minutes.

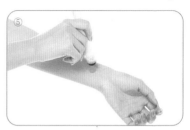

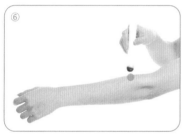

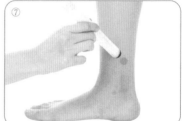

Cupping

Cupping can improve poor blood flow in the neck. When performing this therapy, it is necessary to identify the correct acupoints. If the purple marks from your last cupping session have not yet disappeared, it is not advisable to repeat the treatment. Each cupping session should not be too long. You can use either the fire cupping (a flame is applied to the inside of the cup to remove oxygen) or other convenient cups such as air pump cups. Do not shower until 2 hours after a session. Turn your neck frequently, avoid spicy food, and refrain from keeping a static posture.

Cupping Methods

❶ Place a cup on the Dazhui point for 5 to 10 minutes.

❷ Place a cup on the Fengmen point for 5 to 10 minutes.

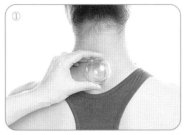

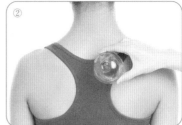

(Remove clothes. The picture is only for illustration.)

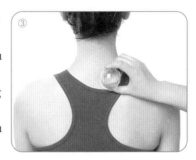

❸ Place a cup on the Dazhu point for 5 to 10 minutes.

❹ Place a cup on the Jianjing point for 5 to 10 minutes.

❺ Place a cup on the Jianyu point for 5 to 10 minutes.

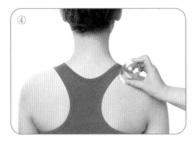

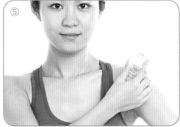

Cupping Points

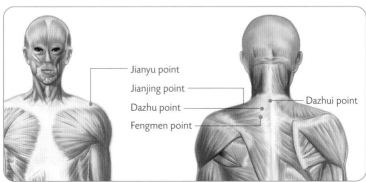

Jianyu point

Jianjing point

Dazhu point

Fengmen point

Dazhui point

Water Therapy

Water therapy can relieve stiffness in the neck muscles. During a session, the water temperature should not be too high, and the hot water should be changed frequently. After a session, wipe yourself dry immediately, and avoid wind exposure. At the same time, having sufficient sleep and taking nutritional supplements is equally important.

Water Therapy Methods

❶ Soak towels in warm water (about 50 ℃), and fold them into small squares. After wringing them dry, place them directly on the back of the neck, occiput, back, shoulder, and other painful and uncomfortable places. Then, dry the areas quickly by wiping them with a dry towel. This is to prevent moisture from taking away heat from the skin.

❷ Pour hot water (about 50 ℃) into a basin, and then soak the affected side of the upper limb in the basin. For the parts that cannot be immersed in the basin, wrap them with towels and pour hot water on them to soak them, or rub them repeatedly with a towel. Rub slowly to avoid damaging the skin. Change the hot water from time to time to maintain a suitable temperature.

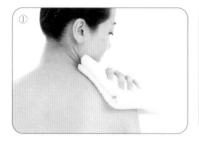 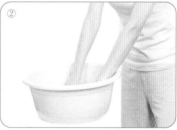

❸ Fill the bathtub with warm water (about 40 ℃). The patient lies on the back, immersing the back of the neck with the rest of the body in water (a damp hot towel can be used as a pillow to support the back of the head and neck). While soaking, massage and rub the affected part at the same time to enhance the curative effect. During water therapy, if the patient experiences dizziness, palpitations, shortness of breath, or fatigue, stop the treatment immediately. The room temperature should not be too low during water therapy.

❹ Pour warm water (about 50 ℃) into a foot bath basin or wooden bucket. The patient sits on a stool and immerses the feet. While soaking, rub the feet together to improve blood circulation. To maintain the water temperature, change the hot water from time to time. If the lower limbs are not sensitive, check the water temperature to prevent scalding.

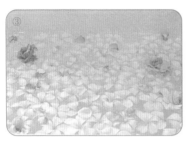 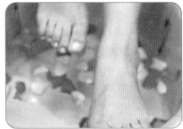

Exercise

When performing daily neck exercise, you should correct bad posture, avoid cold and humid environments, and be persistent. At the same time, make sure you get enough sleep, eat regularly, and avoid keeping still for too long.

Exercise Methods

❶ Stand naturally. The outer edges of both feet should be at the same width as the shoulders, and your hands should droop naturally. Inhale, and turn your head to the left with your peripheral vision towards the edge of the left shoulder. Feel the stretching of the ligament on the right side of your neck. Hold this posture and breathe in and out naturally, three times. Inhale, return your head to the center, breathe, and relax.

❷ Inhale, and turn your head to the right so your peripheral vision is towards the edge of your right shoulder. Feel the stretch of the left ligament of your neck. Hold this posture and breathe in and out naturally, three times. Inhale, return your head to the center, breathe, and relax.

❸ Exhale and bend your head forward with your chin close to the clavicle. Stretch the back of your cervical spine. Hold this posture and breathe in and out naturally, twice. Inhale, return your head to the center, breathe, and relax.

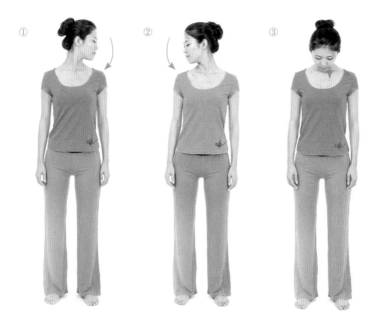

❹ Inhale, raise your head back in a controlled way, and feel the compression of your cervical spine. Hold the posture and breathe in and out naturally twice (reduce to once if you get dizzy when looking up). Inhale, slowly return your head to the center, breathe, and relax.

❺ Exhale, tilt your head to your left shoulder, and push your right hand out horizontally to the right with your fingertips pointing upward. You'll feel a strong stretch of the ligament on the right side of your neck and the muscle of your arm. Hold this posture, and breathe in and out naturally twice. Inhale, return your head and arms to their original positions, breathe, and relax.

❻ Exhale, tilt your head to your right shoulder, and push your left hand out horizontally to the left with your fingertips pointing upward. You'll feel a strong stretch of the left ligament of your neck and the muscles of your arms. Hold this posture and breathe in and out naturally twice. Inhale, return your head and arms to their original position, breathe, and relax.

④
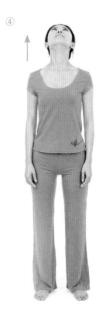

⑤
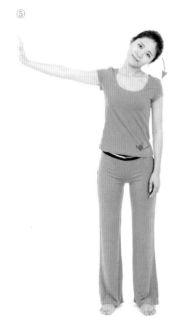

⑥
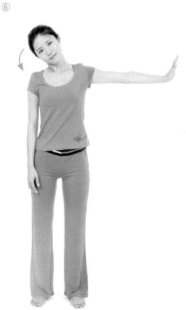

Chapter Three
Treatments to Relieve Shoulder Pain

The shoulder is a part of the body that is easily overlooked. Unless they experience pain, people often do not realize that they need to look after their shoulders. Baring your shoulders in summer, exposing them to a blowing fan during sleep, and staying in one position for a prolonged period can lead to shoulder pain. Sometimes, the pain will be relieved just by moving your muscles and bones. However, if the pain has accumulated over a period of time, it will become a hidden hazard for shoulder problems. Therefore, we should pay more attention to looking after our shoulders.

1. Understanding Shoulder Pain

Cervical spondylosis, cholecystitis, gallstones, and even angina pectoris may cause varying degrees of shoulder pain. Not all shoulder pain is caused by frozen shoulder. It should be identified and treated in a timely manner.

Knowing about Your Shoulder Joints
The shoulder is the most mobile part of the body, but it is also the least stable. To maintain the stability of the shoulder joint, the surrounding muscles and ligaments have to support it.

A large number of muscles surround the shoulder joint, which is of great significance in maintaining its stability. However, there are fewer muscles at the lower front part of the joint. The joint capsule is the most relaxed, so it is the weakest point in terms of joint stability.

The shoulder joint—a typical ball and socket—is composed of the glenoid of the humeral head and scapula. The glenoid is small and shallow, with the glenoid labrum at the edge. The tendon of the long head of the biceps brachii passes through the joint capsule, while the coracohumeral ligament, coracoacromial ligament, and other tendons outside the joint capsule strengthen its stability. The only part that has no ligament and tendon reinforcement is the lower part of the capsule, so it is the weakest. The sizes of the articular surface vary greatly, and the capsule is weak and loose. There are around three ligaments and tendons connecting it, and the triangular deltoid muscle is wrapped around the three sides of the acromion.

Causes of Shoulder Pain

Shoulder pain accounts for a certain proportion of shoulder problems. The main causes of shoulder pain are as follows:

•Long-term desk-bound work or excessive use of computer and mobile phone. Maintaining a fixed posture for a long time will lead to joint stiffness and pain.

•Overstraining of the shoulder. Strain can lead to a pulled shoulder muscle.

•Attack of external pathogens. Wind, Cold and Dampness[1] can lead to poor blood circulation, resulting in inflammation.

Nowadays, shoulder muscle strain—the predecessor of frozen shoulder—is a common ailment. Muscle strain happens before any lesion occurs in the shoulder. Strain happens when a fixed posture is maintained for a long time, damaging soft tissues such as muscles, tendons, nerves, and blood vessels. Once the shoulder is strained, the patient will experience tenderness, numbness, and even severe pain. The average time for a static muscle injury to occur is about two hours. After two hours,

---

[1]Refer to page 19 about Wind and Cold. Dampness is related more to the rainy season, geographical areas with high humidity, and working environments that are close to water. It is related to the spleen system.

injury will occur, and may accumulate. If you remain in the same posture for a long time, there is a high likelihood of developing frozen shoulder. Like cervical spondylosis, shoulder muscle strain is becoming a serious problem among younger people with very similar occupations. Almost all of them are either white-collar office workers or drivers. Modern working styles and living habits also contribute to shoulder pain. For example, many people do not sit correctly, tilting their shoulder blades. Over time, these muscles will suffer from strain that will increase the risk of an attack of frozen shoulder in the future.

Middle aged people, especially those around the age of 50, are prone to pain in the shoulder joints. In the early stages for most people, soring pain is mainly experienced in the shoulders, and becomes more severe in the evening or in winter. On these occasions, shoulder movement becomes less flexible, and patients begin to experience stiffness. Gradually, the pain will begin to affect the neck and upper limbs. Shoulder movements become limited, and even simple actions like lifting the arm will become difficult, such as stretching the arms, combing hair, taking off clothes, and putting hands on hips. Most people around the age of 50 will experience a sharp decrease in hormone levels. This reduces the secretion of synovial fluid in the shoulder joints, and lowers the degree of lubrication, resulting in pain. After developing this condition, if they suffer an injury, Wind, Cold, or over-exhaustion, the shoulder joints will be prone to muscle and ligament bleeding, edema, and inflammation, which will eventually lead to stiffness and adhesion of the shoulder joint and its surrounding tissues.

2. Common Acupoints for Relieving Shoulder Pain

Although the conditions that lead to shoulder pain are many, there are differences if we analyze them. For example, pain caused by simple frozen shoulder is only limited to the shoulder, while pain caused by cervical spine problems is often accompanied by discomfort or pain in the lower neck, and numbness of fingers. Patients with angina pectoris will also experience tightness in the retrosternal or precordial area. Patients should carefully analyze their etiology before carrying out massage therapy to avoid delay in receiving the correct treatment.

Six Main Acupoints

Jianzhen point: located on the lower part of the back of the shoulder joint, and 1 cun above the posterior axillary fold. The Jianzhen point is used to treat frozen shoulder when combined with the Jianyu and Jianliao points.

Dazhu point: located at the junction of the neck and back, this is a good choice for the treatment of neck-shoulder bone and joint problems.

Jianzhongshu point: located 2 cun away from the underside of the spinous process of the seventh cervical vertebra. It is connected to the neck at the top, the back at the bottom, and the shoulder at the side. Massage it to alleviate discomfort in the shoulder, neck, and back.

Jianjing point: located at the midpoint of the connecting line between the Dazhui point and the acromion. Press it to get rid of tension and stiffness in the shoulder and neck muscles quickly.

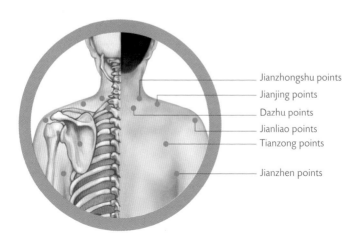

Jianzhongshu points
Jianjing points
Dazhu points
Jianliao points
Tianzong points
Jianzhen points

Jianliao point: raise your arm horizontally. At the depression behind the acromion, which can be used to treat shoulder and back pain.

Tianzong point: extend your hand across your neck to the scapula on the opposite side of your shoulder. The point where the pulp of your middle finger rests is the Tianzong point. It's one of the most commonly used points for the treatment of back-shoulder injury and frozen shoulder.

Massage Tips
If you have a frozen shoulder, ask someone to apply an oil lubricant around the Jianjing point, and then use an ox horn scraper to glide or scrape repeatedly in an outward direction around the shoulder area. If there is obvious swelling or pain in some parts, a little more force can be applied.

3. Massage Methods for Shoulder Pain

Prolonged periods in sedentary or incorrect sitting postures will lead to shoulder pain. The root of the problem is a lack of *qi* and blood[1]. Massage therapy can clear congestion in the *qi* and blood, and can maintain the health of the shoulders and neck. When using a computer or using your mobile phone, it is important to move your neck and shoulders every 40 minutes.

Frozen Shoulder

The main symptom of frozen shoulder is gradual pain in the shoulder, which gets worse at night. It is usually related to bad

---

[1] *Qi* is the most fundamental substance of the human body. It is the energy or life-process that flows in and around all of us. Blood—a nutritious red fluid that flows in the vessels—is one of the essential substances that make up the human body and maintain life and activity.

living habits. It is essential to maintain good habits that include, exercising regularly, getting enough sleep, and avoiding being in a prolonged fixed posture. To relieve pain, massage therapy should be carried out alongside joint function exercises, in combination with therapy methods such as moxibustion or *gua sha* scraping.

During an attack, massage should be performed once in the morning and once in the evening, with each session lasting 20 minutes. During the recovery period, massage once a day for 15 minutes. For normal healthcare, massage 3 times a week, for 15 minutes each time.

Massage Points

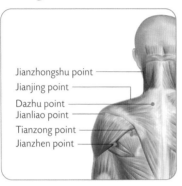

Jianzhongshu point

Jianjing point

Dazhu point

Jianliao point

Tianzong point

Jianzhen point

Massage Methods

❶ Sit the patient up. Stand at the posterolateral side from the affected shoulder joint. Using the rolling technique, move hand back and forth alternately around the shoulder for 1 to 3 minutes, so as to alleviate the spasm and adhesion of muscles, ligaments and other soft tissues.

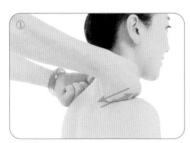

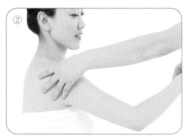

❷ First, push-press the front and back of the patient's shoulder joint with palms. Then, use the thumb and the other four fingers to grasp and pinch or press the Dazhu, Jianjing, Tianzong, Jianzhongshu, Jianliao, and Jianzhen points for 1 to 3 minutes to dredge the meridians and collaterals, promote *qi*, and relieve pain.

❸ Use the palm to push-press from the spinous process of the first to seventh thoracic vertebrae on the patient's back, to the parts around the shoulders on both sides, or rub the parts above with the hypothenar[1] of the palm. Then use the palm roots and thumbs, press and knead the medial edge of the patient's scapula on both shoulders and the anterior, posterior, lateral, and axilla parts of the shoulder joints.

❹ Gently pat the area around the patient's shoulder, and rub and knead their arm from top to bottom.

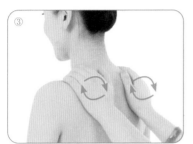
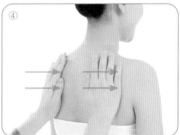

Shoulder Muscle Strain

The symptoms are soreness, numbness, and even severe pain in the shoulder. This is usually related to the vigorous movement of the upper limbs. If you experience these symptoms, you should rest immediately and seek medication or physiotherapy. Strenuous exercises of the upper limbs must be avoided. Instead, stretching exercises should be done regularly, alongside moxibustion and other methods of alleviating pain.

During an attack, massage should be performed once in the morning and once in the evening, with each session lasting 15 minutes. During the recovery period, massage once a day for 10 minutes. For normal healthcare, massage 3 times a week, for 10 minutes each time.

---

[1] The group of muscles that control the movement of the little finger.

Massage Points

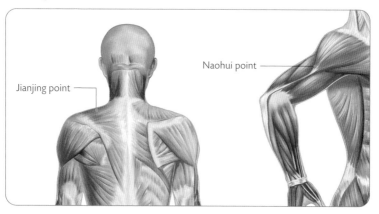

Massage Methods

❶ Sit the patient up. Stand on the posterolateral side of his/her affected shoulder joint, grasp the patient's shoulder, and press the Jianjing point with the thumb. This can alleviate shoulder pain.

❷ The patient stands and presses the Naohui point with the finger pulp for 1 to 3 minutes. This is very effective at relieving pain in the upper arm.

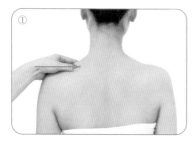
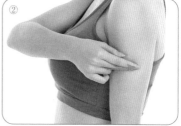

❸ Hold the patient's shoulder with one hand and his/her wrist with the other hand. Make a rotation movement centered on the shoulder joint, ranging from small to large, applying pressure that is within the patient's tolerance level.

❹ Hold the patient's wrist with both hands and swing the upper limbs up, down, left, and right respectively for about 5 minutes.

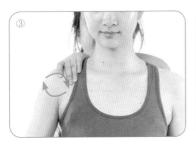
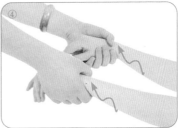

Sore Shoulder

Sore shoulders are related to bad living habits. Symptoms include a feeling of tenderness in the shoulder. In severe cases, a sufferer can experience intense pain. You should avoid being in a fixed posture for a long time. Change your sitting posture, get enough sleep, and do more stretching exercise. If you feel discomfort in your shoulder, you should rest immediately and get a timely massage, alongside scraping, moxibustion, and other methods of alleviating pain.

During an attack, massage should be performed once in the morning and once in the evening, with each session lasting 15 minutes. During the recovery period, massage once a day for 10 minutes. For normal healthcare, massage twice a week, for 10 minutes each time.

Massage Methods

❶ Flex the joints of fingers and palm, then with the wrist joint as the source of flexion, rotate the forearm and roll the back of hand back and forth continuously on the affected part of the patient.

❷ Clamp the affected part of the patient with the palms of both hands. Rub-knead rapidly in the same direction with relative force, or in a clockwise direction. When rubbing, the force applied should be uniform and moderate, and the action should be gentle and even.

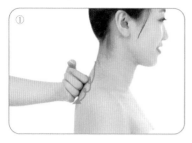

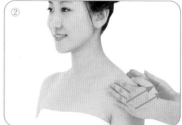

❸ Use the thumb, palm, or fist to exert pressure on the painful shoulder. Press and move in a straight-line or arch along a single direction.

❹ Exert relative force with the thumb and the other four fingers to grasp and pinch the lesion. Or, use the force from a "3-finger grasp" formed by your thumb, index finger, and middle finger on the shoulder and neck to alleviate pain.

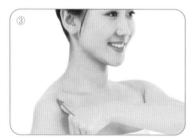

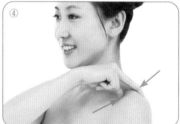

4. Other Methods for Shoulder Pain

In addition to acupoint massage, you can also use methods such as moxibustion, cupping, *gua sha* scraping, and exercise to alleviate shoulder pain.

Moxibustion

During moxibustion, the moxa stick should not come into direct contact with the skin, and each session should not be too long. Moxibustion should be avoided if you are running a fever. Refrain from being in a prolonged fixed position. During the treatment period, make sure you get enough sleep and take proper exercise.

During an attack, carry out moxibustion therapy once in the morning and once in the evening, with each session lasting 25 minutes. During the recovery period, do it once a day for 10 minutes. For normal healthcare, carry out the treatment twice a week, for 10 minutes each time.

Moxibustion Points

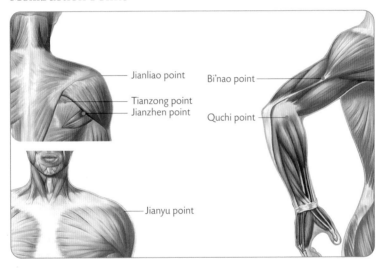

Moxibustion Methods

❶ Ignite the moxa stick. Place it 1.5 to 3 cm away from the Jianliao point, and hold it there for 3 to 5 minutes.

❷ Ignite the moxa stick. Place it 1.5 to 3 cm away from the Jianyu point, and hold it there for 3 to 5 minutes.

❸ Ignite the moxa stick. Place it 1.5 to 3 cm away from the Tianzong point, and hold it there for 3 to 5 minutes.

❹ Ignite the moxa stick. Place it 1.5 to 3 cm away from the Bi'nao point, and hold it there for 3 to 5 minutes.

❺ Ignite the moxa stick. Place it 1.5 to 3 cm away from the Jianzhen point, and hold it there for 3 to 5 minutes.

❻ Ignite the moxa stick. Place it 1.5 to 3 cm away from the Quchi point, and hold it there for 3 to 5 minutes.

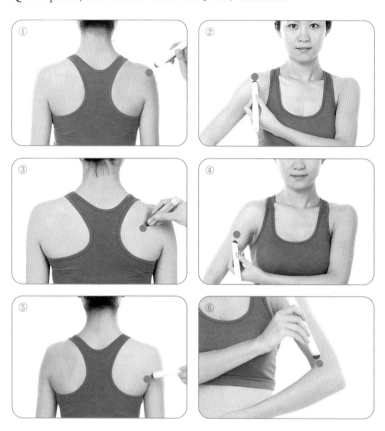

Cupping

Cupping can improve blood flow in the body. When performing this therapy, it is necessary to find the right acupoints. If the purple marks from the last cupping session have not disappeared, it is not advisable to repeat the treatment yet. Each session should not last too long, and you can use either the fire or air pump method. Do not take a shower until 2 hours after each cupping session. In your daily life, you should relax your body, avoid strenuous exercise, and maintain air circulation in your environment.

Cupping Points

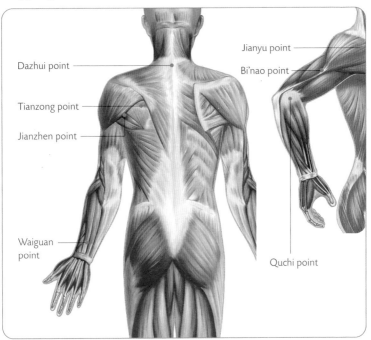

Cupping Methods

❶ Put the cup on the Waiguan point for 5 to 10 minutes.

❷ Put the cup on the Tianzong point for 5 to 10 minutes.

❸ Put the cup on the Dazhui point for 5 to 10 minutes.

❹ Put the cup on the Jianzhen point for 5 to 10 minutes.

❺ Put the cup on the Bi'nao point for 5 to 10 minutes.

❻ Put the cup on the Jianyu point for 5 to 10 minutes.

❼ Put the cup on the Quchi point for 5 to 10 minutes.

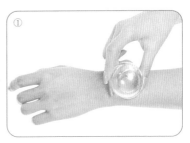

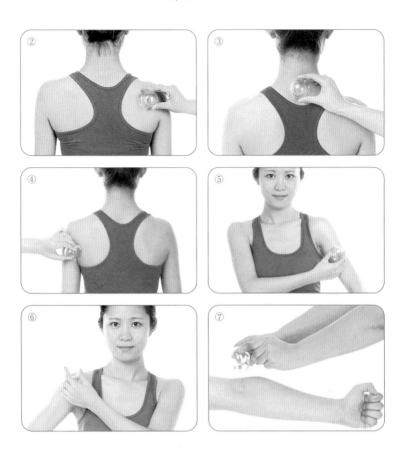

Gua Sha Scraping

During a *gua sha* scraping session, the duration and the pressure applied are based on the patient's level of tolerance. After scraping, drink warm water, stay out of the wind, and keep warm. Do not shower until 3 hours after a scraping session. In your daily life, you should maintain a healthy diet, take proper exercise, and refrain from maintaining a fixed posture.

One of the methods of *gua sha* is flat scraping, which uses the flat edge of the scraping tool. Hold the scraping tool at an angle of about 15 degrees to the skin, and scrape the area evenly in a straight line in one direction. During an attack, scrape once every alternate day, for 10 minutes each time. During the recovery period, scrape twice a week, for 5 minutes each time. For daily healthcare, scrape once a week, for 5 minutes each time.

Scraping Points

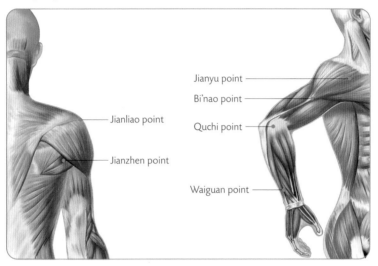

Jianyu point

Bi'nao point

Jianliao point

Quchi point

Jianzhen point

Waiguan point

Scraping Method

❶ Use the flat scraping method, increase the intensity, and scrape the Jianyu point downwards from top to bottom repeatedly until red marks (*sha*) appear.

❷ Use the flat scraping method, increase the intensity, and scrape the Jianzhen point downwards from top to bottom repeatedly until red marks appear.

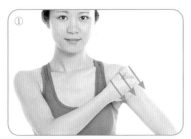

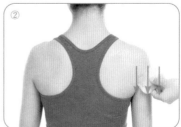

❸ Use the flat scraping method, increase the intensity, and scrape the Jianliao point outwards from inside to outside, repeatedly until red marks appear.

❹ Use the flat scraping method, scrape the Waiguan point downwards from top to bottom repeatedly until red marks appear.

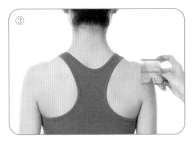
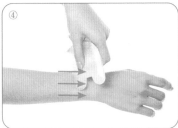

❺ Use the flat scraping method, and scrape the Quchi point downwards from top to bottom repeatedly until red marks appear.

❻ Use the flat scraping method, increase the intensity, and scrape the Bi'nao point downwards from top to bottom repeatedly until red marks appear.

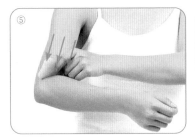
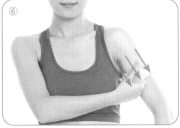

Exercise

When performing shoulder exercise, it is important not to overdo it, and to maintain correct posture and exercise daily. At the same time, make sure you keep warm, get enough sleep, have a healthy diet, and avoid maintaining a fixed posture. During an attack period, exercise once a day, for 15 minutes each time; in the recovery period, exercise once a day, for 10 minutes each time; for daily healthcare, exercise 3 times a week, for 10 minutes each time.

Exercise Methods

❶ Relax both shoulders, flex your elbows, with your arms below your shoulders and hands on shoulders. Then, taking the shoulder as the axis, first draw a small circle, and then increase the range of the circle gradually. Do this once a day, 10 times clockwise, then 10 times counterclockwise.

❷ Stand upright and relax. Place your right hand on your left shoulder and gently knead it 20 to 30 times. Then, put your left hand on your right shoulder and knead it gently 20 to 30 times. Do this until you feel a slight warmth in your shoulders.

❸ Stand with your arms drooping naturally. Breathe evenly. When inhaling, stretch both arms forward gradually and lift them up as high as possible. When exhaling, put your arms down, keeping them straight, and swing them behind you as

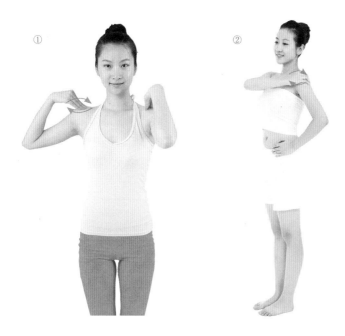

far back as possible. Swing continuously 10 to 15 times. Then, return to your original position and take a break. The above actions can be repeated 1 to 3 times.

❹ Stand with your feet apart at shoulder width, with your arms drooping to the sides. Breathe evenly. Bend your knees. Move your left hand from your left thigh, past the lower abdomen, and then your chest as if drawing a circle upwards to the left. Your waist should turn to the left simultaneously with this action, with your body weight gradually shifting to rest on your left foot, then back to the original standing position. Then, repeat this action with your right hand but in the opposite direction; first from the right thigh, passing the lower abdomen and chest, with your waist simultaneously turning to the right, and your body weight gradually shifting to rest on the right foot. The above actions can be repeated 20 to 30 times.

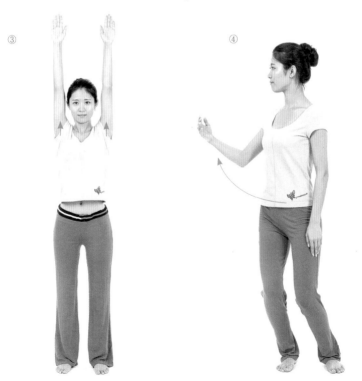

③   ④

Chapter Four
Treatments to Relieve Lower Back Pain

Many people will experience lower back pain if they stay in a fixed position for a long time. The lumbar spine bears more than 60% of the weight of the human body, and is often in a state of tension and fatigue. Strain and degeneration begins to occur in the absence of enough sleep and exercise. In normal physical activities, the lumbar spine does not injure easily. However, once aching begins, this is a warning sign that the body is suffering, and that appropriate care and attention should be given.

1. Understanding Lower Back Pain

The lumbar region is the strongest part of the spine. Serving as the base for the whole spinal network, the lumbar spine and sacral spine have thick vertebral bodies and strong muscles. The sacral spine and pelvis form a force converter that distributes body weight equally between the two legs. Lumbosacral strain, which is a common ailment among the elderly, is an accumulated injury of the ligaments and joint capsules.

Knowing about the Lumbosacral Vertebrae
The lumbosacral vertebrae include the lumbar vertebrae and sacral vertebrae. The sacral vertebrae and the left and right hip bones form the pelvis. In the mechanical structure of spine, the lumbosacral vertebrae are base, and have strong muscles and thick vertebral bodies. Their most important function is to support the body and maintain movement.

The lumbar section of the spine bears the most weight, and the posterior part of the upper lumbar spine is slightly sunken.

The cross section of lumbar vertebrae L1–L2 is shaped like a kidney, and the transition in lumbar vertebrae L3 or L4 is an oval. The middle of the posterior edge of the lumbar vertebrae L5 is raised slightly higher than the two sides, and the vertebral body is shaped like an olive.

Causes of Lumbar Pain

It is a commonly held belief that when you have lower back pain, you should sit down, as it is assumed that sitting is resting. In reality, this assumption is wrong. Research has proved that when we sit, especially with an incorrect posture, the lumbar intervertebral disc is under the greatest pressure. With the right posture, the pressure in the lumbar intervertebral disc is six times that of the supine position. An incorrect sitting posture, such as leaning forward for a long time, will cause the pressure in the lumbar intervertebral disc to soar to 11 times that of the supine position. Sitting actually increases the burden on the lumbar spine. Sitting for prolonged periods also means that your entire body weight is on the lumbosacral vertebrae, leading to tension and fatigue of the lumbar and abdominal muscles.

So what is the correct posture? According to the principles of biomechanics, any posture that keeps the spine in a normal physiological curve is correct. Any posture that does not conform to the normal physiological curve, or causes damage to it, is wrong. To avoid bodily fatigue, work on keeping an even weight distribution and maintain balance. This depends mainly on a normal physiological spinal curve.

Because the lumbar spine is at the base of the trunk, the lumbar intervertebral disc has to be stronger, thicker, and larger than other intervertebral discs. The reasons for lumbar pain are many, such as:

• Being sedentary: spending prolonged periods in a fixed posture.

• Bending over doing housework: a lot more pressure is put on the lower back.

• Obesity: affecting the normal physiological curvature and spinal stress point.

Checking Your Lumbar Health

When a problem with the lumbosacral vertebrae arises, it is usually accompanied by some unconscious habits. Do you do the following things?

• Always carrying or holding things on one particular side, and feeling uncomfortable doing so on the other side.

• In your most natural posture when standing at ease, the leg supporting your weight often feels slightly shorter and stronger than the other extended leg. When sitting down with one leg crossing over the other, or lying down, this leg is often the one that is placed on top of the other leg. Other postures make you feel awkward. When walking forward, this leg often steps out later.

• When wearing trousers, you notice that one leg is longer than the other.

• When jumping on one leg, you find that it is always more flexible than the other.

• The soles of your shoe wear out at different rates.

2. Common Acupoints for Relieving Lower Back Pain

If you suffer a lesion in your lumbar spine, you will experience stiffness in your lower back in addition to pain, and your range of movement will become smaller. Any activity will aggravate the pain. Symptoms also include weakness and tenderness in the lower and upper back, as well as pain and discomfort, accompanied by dizziness. If you experience pain or numbness in your legs in addition to lower back pain, it usually indicates that your lumbar nerve roots are being compressed. Most cases are caused by health issues such as lumbar disc herniation, lumbar spinal stenosis, or even spinal canal tumors. It may not be merely a simple injury of the lumbar soft tissue.

Twelve Main Acupoints

Yaoshu point: located on the posterior midline, facing the sacral hiatus, Yaoshu is one of the most commonly used points to clear congestion in the Du Meridian[1] and the Zusanyang meridians[2].

Yaoyangguan point: this point is often combined with the Shenshu, Dachangshu, and Baliao points for acupuncture or massage to treat ailments such as lumbosacral pain clinically.

Chengfu points: these points are located at the mid-point of the horizontal line under the buttocks. To relieve ailments such as lower back pain, massage the Chengfu points upward with the pulp of your index finger, middle finger, and ring finger.

Jiaji points: TCM practitioners often select the Jiaji points for acupuncture or massage when treating the spine or related illnesses.

Shenshu points: TCM refers the lower back as "the house of the kidneys." The Shenshu points are an ideal choice for those who want to replenish kidney *qi*, whether through acupuncture or massage.

Dachangshu points: these points can relieve nerve compression in the case of lower back and lower limb pain, numbness, or muscle atrophy.

Huantiao points: for lower back and leg pain, massage from the Huantiao point downward to the Weizhong, Chengshan, and Kunlun points. This will dispel Wind, Cold, Dampness pathogens, and will also relieve pain, relax the tendons, and benefit the joints.

Baliao points: these points are located at the hip and sacrum, connecting the lower back at the top and the lower limbs at the

---

[1] The Du Meridian (also known as the Governing Vessel) is one of the eight extraordinary meridians. The acupoints on the Du Meridian are mainly located on the middle line of the back.

[2] The Zusanyang meridians refer to the Yangming Stomach Meridian of Foot (ST), the Shaoyang Gallbladder Meridian of Foot (GB), and the Taiyang Bladder Meridian of Foot (BL), all of which are among the twelve main meridians of the human body.

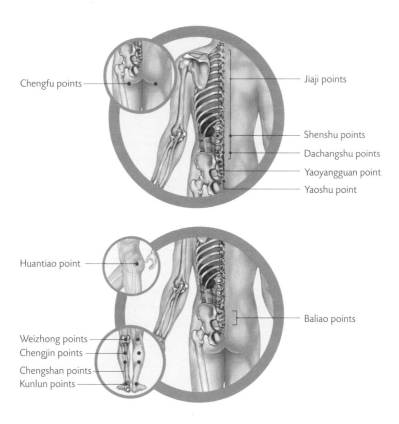

Chengfu points — Jiaji points — Shenshu points — Dachangshu points — Yaoyangguan point — Yaoshu point

Huantiao point — Baliao points

Weizhong points — Chengjin points — Chengshan points — Kunlun points

bottom. Massaging the Baliao points alleviates pain in the lower back, and treats discomfort in the legs and feet.

Chengjin points: massage these points often, as they have the function of dispelling Heat and Dampness in the body and strengthening the lower back and knees.

Kunlun points: applying acupuncture or massage therapy to these points is effective in clearing congestion in the meridians and collaterals, dispersing Cold and relieving pain, promoting *qi*, and improving blood circulation.

Weizhong points: press the Weizhong points with your thumbs repeatedly. These points are suitable for treating all kinds of lower back and knee pain.

Chengshan points: by massaging the Chengshan points, you can dispel the pathogenic factors of the Wind and Cold, promote *yang qi*, and dredge the meridians.

Tips for Lower Back Care

It is not realistic to maintain the correct posture all the time, without slacking off for a moment. Therefore, we need to think of alternative ways to solve this problem. For example, after you've been sitting for an hour or two, do a forward flexion, backward extension, and rotation of the head and upper limbs to alleviate fatigue and enhance muscle tenacity. You can also get up and move around, pour yourself a glass of water, or chat with your colleagues. In other words, refrain from sitting still for too long.

"Backward walking" is a good exercise for people with lower back pain. It is very simple: just walk backwards. Do it daily, once in the morning and once in the evening, for 20 to 30 minutes each time. Take note that when walking backwards, our perception of space will be significantly reduced, making it easy to fall, so walk steadily and do not go too fast. Look behind you from time to time to control your direction. Backward walking can be very effective at alleviating severe lower back pain. Patients with chronic lumbar spine problems should perform backward walking persistently for a prolonged period.

3. Massage Methods for Lower Back Pain

Many lower back ailments will lead to pain, which can be an inconvenience to work and life. This section explains the causes of some lower back issues, and offers massage methods suitable for a variety of symptoms.

Acute Lumbar Sprain

Acute lumbar sprain is an acute tear brought about by excessive traction of the lumbar muscles. This condition is usually related to improper posture or excessive force used when carrying heavy objects. Patients should maintain the correct posture, avoid sitting still for a long time, eat a healthy diet, engage in massage therapy, and exercise appropriately. Other therapeutic pain-relieving treatments can be carried out as well, include *gua sha* scraping and cupping.

During an attack, massage should be performed once in the morning and once in the evening, with each session lasting 20 minutes. During the recovery period, massage once a day for 15 minutes. For normal healthcare, massage twice a week, for 15 minutes each time.

Massage Points

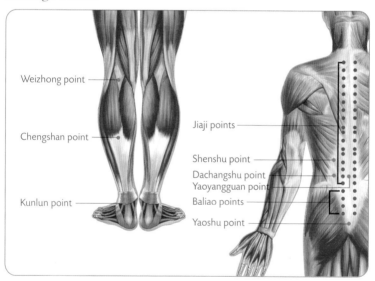

Massage Methods

❶ Put the patient in the prone position on the bed. Rub both palms together until they feel hot; place both palms either side of the patient's lumbar spine, then push and wipe downwards repeatedly until the skin turns red and the temperature rises. This will improve blood circulation in the patient's lumbar spine.

❷ With the patient still in the prone position, use the pulp of both thumbs, or the thenar[1] and hypothenar of the palm to press and knead the sore points along both sides of the lumbar spine muscles. Then massage by following this order: press the Jiaji, Shenshu, Dachangshu, Yaoyangguan, Baliao, Yaoshu points in the lower back and sacrum, and Weizhong, Chengshan, Kunlun points in the lower limbs. This will relieve the spasm in the patient's lumbar muscles.

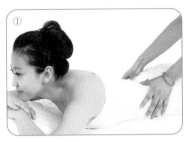
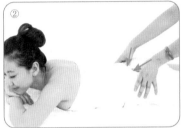

❸ Use the tips of both thumbs to press down deeply on one side of the patient's lumbar ligaments, muscles, and tendons. Then, exerting more force, pluck back and forth perpendicular to the ligaments or muscle fibers, to further relieve tension in the lumbar muscles and ligaments.

❹ With one palm on top of the other hand, place both hands on the patient's lumbosacral joints. First press down several times, then close your five fingers together like a half-clenched fist. Beat repeatedly on the patient's lumbosacral parts to alleviate muscle spasm or correct disorders of the lumbar facet joints.

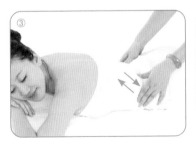
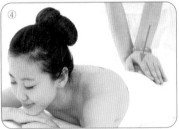

---

[1] The mound formed at the base of the thumb on the palm of the hand by the intrinsic group of muscles of the thumb.

Chronic Lumbar Muscle Strain

This is usually related to fatigue and climate changes in the living environment. The condition recurs over and over, and persists for a long time. If you are a sufferer, avoid overexerting yourself and try not to catch colds. Keep warm, and eat food that nourishes your kidneys. Hot water can be used to shower the affected area. A hot compress treatment alongside therapeutic treatment methods such as moxibustion and cupping can be carried out to relieve pain.

During an attack, massage should be performed once in the morning and once in the evening, with each session lasting 20 minutes. During the recovery period, massage once a day for 20 minutes. For normal healthcare, massage twice a week, for 15 minutes each time.

Massage Points

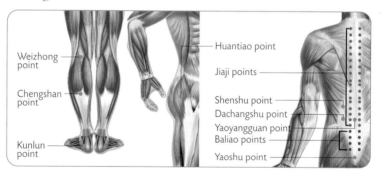

Weizhong point

Chengshan point

Kunlun point

Huantiao point

Jiaji points

Shenshu point

Dachangshu point

Yaoyangguan point

Baliao points

Yaoshu point

Massage Methods

❶ Put the patient in the prone position. Use the root of palm, work along the route of the Taiyang Bladder Meridian of Foot on both sides of the lower back (refer to the orange lines in the figure at the top left on page 83) from top to bottom, exerting increasing pressure. Press and knead to the lumbosacral part repeatedly.

❷ Use the pulp of both thumbs to press and knead the points of the lower back and sacrum in this order: Jiaji, Shenshu, Dachangshu, Yaoyangguan, Baliao, and Yaoshu points. You

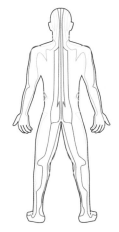

Main meridians on the back of the body.

can also press the Huantiao, Weizhong, Chenshan, and the Kunlun points on the lower limbs. According to clinical observations, it is a good sign when soreness, distention, numbness, and heaviness occur at the acupoints during massage.

❸ Use the thumb and the other four fingers to lift and grasp on the patient's lumbar muscles, first move up and then down. Increase pressure gradually, massaging first on the healthy side, then moving to the affected side. Then with the side of the back of your half-clenched fists, gently tap the patient's lower back and sacrum area. This can also be done with tools such as bamboo strips.

❹ Ask the patient to lie on their back and relax their muscles. Stand at their heels and hold the two ankle joints separately with your hands. Pull them in a downward direction, and shake the lower back muscles rapidly several times.

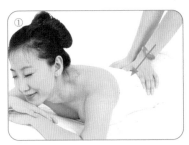

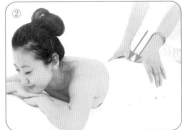

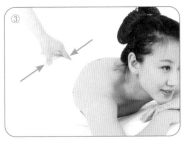

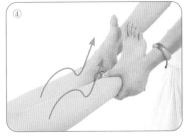

Lumbar Disc Herniation

Normally, between each vertebra of the human spine is an intervertebral disc, composed of a nucleus pulposus and a fibrous ring, which acts as a cushion. When the spine is subjected to longitudinal impact, the disc expands outward to cushion the pressure and absorb the shock. This prevents impact and injury to the body when walking, bouncing, or running. The intervertebral discs play a very important role, especially in protecting the fragile brain. The constant shape-changing of the discs can also increase the mobility of the spine, allowing it to move flexibly in all directions.

Lumbar disc herniation causes lumbar pain and numbness in one or both lower limbs. This condition is usually related to a lesion or injury to one of the lumbar discs. If this happens to you, avoid lifting heavy objects. Get plenty of rest, exercise regularly, and build up your immunity. Hot water can be used on the affected area in the shower.

During an attack, massage should be performed once in the morning and once in the evening, with each session lasting 20 minutes. During the recovery period, massage once a day for 20 minutes. For normal healthcare, massage twice a week, for 15 minutes each time.

Massage Points

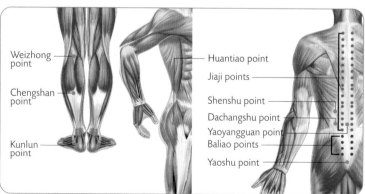

Weizhong point

Chengshan point

Kunlun point

Huantiao point

Jiaji points

Shenshu point

Dachangshu point

Yaoyangguan point

Baliao points

Yaoshu point

Massage Methods

❶ Put the patient in sitting position. Sit behind him/her, and push and knead repeatedly with the tip of thumb or the tip of elbow on the aching points around the lumbar lesion. Then, applying deep pressure, press with your palm or fingertips on the Jiaji, Shenshu, Dachangshu, Yaoyangguan, Baliao, and Yaoshu points on the patient's lower back and sacrum. Press for about 1 minute on each acupoint.

❷ Get the patient to lean back and relax the tensed psoas muscles. This time, the focus will be on the main part of the lesion—every intervertebral space of the lumbar spine. First, perform a forward-push manipulation on each one of them, followed by a relaxing press and knead manipulation. Spend about 1 to 2 minutes for each manipulation.

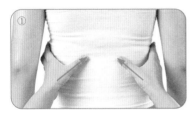
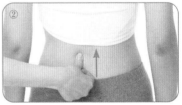

❸ Clench the fists, and knock rhythmically along both sides of the lumbar spine to the lumbosacral joint. You can also rub your hands together, and place your hot palms directly on both sides of the patient's lumbar spine, where the Jiaji points are, and rub back and forth.

❹ After treating the lower back, use the pulp of thumbs to knead and press the Huantiao points on the hip, the Weizhong points on the back of the knee, and the Chengshan and Kunlun points on the lower leg for 1 to 3 minutes.

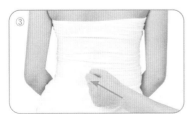
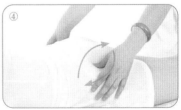

Lumbar Spinal Stenosis

Sometimes, after walking a certain distance, your lower back and legs may begin to feel sore, numb, and painful—a condition known as claudication. It can gradually worsen, making it difficult to continue. After having a rest, either squatting or sitting for a while, the symptoms seem to lessen or disappear, and you can continue with your walk. The above symptoms may appear again on other occasions after you have walked about the same distance or the same length of time. This intermittent claudication is a typical symptom of lumbar spinal stenosis, and is usually related to the degenerative diseases of the spine that occur in middle-aged and elderly people. If early symptoms appear, use this method to alleviate intermittent claudication: lie on your back on the bed, hold your knees with both hands, and get up. Do this exercise 50 to 100 times a day. Make sure you get enough rest, avoid stress, maintain a healthy diet, and correct any spinal problems.

During an attack, massage should be performed once in the morning and once in the evening, with each session lasting 20 minutes. During the recovery period, massage once a day for 15 minutes. For normal healthcare, massage twice a week, for 15 minutes each time.

Massage Points

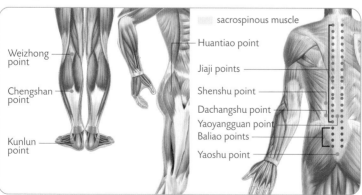

Weizhong point

Chengshan point

Kunlun point

sacrospinous muscle

Huantiao point

Jiaji points

Shenshu point

Dachangshu point

Yaoyangguan point

Baliao points

Yaoshu point

Massage Methods

❶ Put the patient in the prone position. Use either the thenar and hypothenar of palm or the tip of thumb to successively press the Jiaji, Shenshu, Yaoyangguan, Dachangshu, Baliao, and Yaoshu points in the lower back and sacrum, as well as the Huantiao, Weizhong, Chengshan, and Kunlun points in the lower limbs.

❷ With the patient still in the prone position, use the pulp of both thumbs to push-knead the sacrospinous muscle, on both sides of the lumbar spine for 1 to 3 minutes.

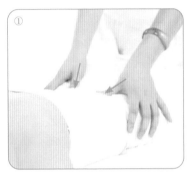
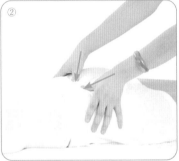

❸ Place your palm on the patient's lumbosacral joint and press it down continuously for 30 seconds.

❹ The patient clenches the fists, and gently strikes repeatedly on the afflicted parts of the lumbar spine, the sacrum, and tailbone. This can also be done with other massage tools.

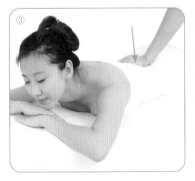
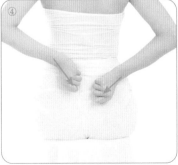

Lumbar Spondylolisthesis

This is usually related to structural abnormalities caused by aging to the lumbar spine due to excessive mechanical stresses. During an attack, be sure to take bed rest. Any activities that add burden to the lower back should be strictly avoided. On normal days, remember to rest, maintain a healthy diet, exercise appropriately, keep weight off your back, and avoid over-exhaustion.

During an attack, massage should be performed once in the morning and once in the evening, with each session lasting 20 minutes. During the recovery period, massage once a day for 15 minutes. For normal healthcare, massage twice a week, for 15 minutes each time.

Massage Methods

❶ Put the patient in the prone position. Stand on one side, and gently press and knead both sides of their lower back, from top to bottom. Repeat this action 3 to 5 times. Do not use too much pressure.

❷ Put the patient in the supine position. Hold their feet with both your hands. Bend their knees and push them towards their head. His/her body will be bent and hips away from the bed. Then, use left palm to press on the patient's abdomen, and with your right elbow on the popliteal fossa[1] of the patient's lower limbs to form the calf and the thigh in 90°, push them towards patient's head.

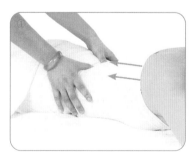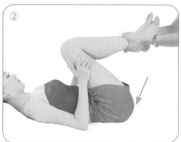

❸ Ask the patient to take the prone position. Hold their knee with one hand and slowly lift it up. Press the other hand tightly on the affected part of the lower back. When the lower back is extended to the maximum, push your hands gently in the opposite direction. This method is more effective for people suffering from backward spondylolysis of the lumbar spine. Do not use brute force.

❹ Ask the patient to lie on their back, bending their knees and hips. With one hand pressing their knee towards their chest; with the other hand holding the patient's hips, roll the patient back and forth in this position 20 times.

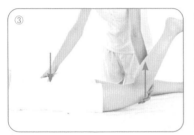
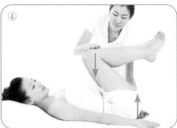

Piriformis Syndrome

This is usually related to compression of the sciatic nerve and inflammation. Patients should rest well, avoid excessive exercise, reduce the burden on the lower back, eat healthily, and use methods such as moxibustion and cupping to alleviate discomfort.

During an attack, massage should be performed once in the morning and once in the evening, with each session lasting 15 minutes. During the recovery period, massage once a day for 15 minutes. For normal healthcare, massage twice a week, for 10 minutes each time.

---

[1] The diamond-shaped space behind the knee joint.

Massage Points

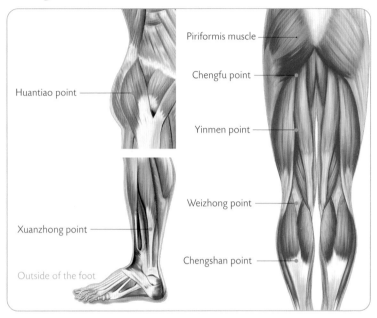

Piriformis muscle

Chengfu point

Huantiao point

Yinmen point

Weizhong point

Xuanzhong point

Chengshan point

Outside of the foot

Massage Methods

❶ Put the patient in the prone position. Stand beside him/her and press and knead the affected area on the buttocks with the root of palm, increasing the pressure and focusing mainly on relaxing the local muscles. Repeat this massage technique for about 5 minutes. On the patient's body surface area where the piriformis muscle[1] is located, use both your hands to pluck 5 to 10 times from the outside to the inside, with intense pressure, at the patient's tolerance level.

❷ Place one hand on the other hand and press and knead the patient's lower back, as well as Huantiao, Chengfu, Yinmen,

---

[1] The piriformis muscle is located at the posterior of the buttocks and starts from the anterior of the sacrum, runs outward, passing through the greater sciatic foramen to reach the hip, and ends at the greater trochanter of the femur.

Weizhong, Chengshan, and Xuanzhong points. Apply moderate pressure, according to the patient's tolerance level.

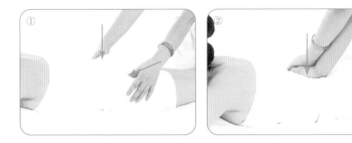

❸ Put the patient in the supine position. Stand on the side where the affected area is. Hold the knee of the affected side with one hand and the ankle with the other. Rotate clockwise and counterclockwise 3 times each.

❹ The patient uses the root of palm to press and knead the affected part for 2 to 3 minutes, until the area feels warm and comfortable.

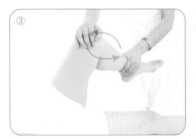
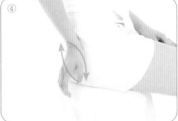

Ankylosing Spondylitis

The early signs of ankylosing spondylitis are mild symptoms throughout the whole body. This is usually related to the main lesion area of chronic spinal disease. Appropriate exercise or painkillers can alleviate it. Patients should seek early diagnosis and early treatment, and maintain an optimistic attitude. Proper rest and a healthy diet are also important in daily life.

During an attack, massage should be performed once in the morning and once in the evening, with each session lasting 20 minutes. During the recovery period, massage once a day for 15 minutes. For normal healthcare, massage twice a week, for 10 minutes each time.

Massage Points

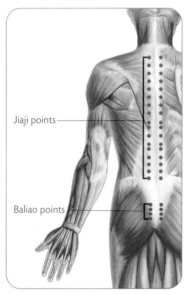

Jiaji points

Baliao points

Massage Methods

❶ Put the patient in the prone position. With both hands, knead and pinch from top to bottom along both sides of the spine, increasing the pressure according to the patient's tolerance level and until redness begin to form around the local area.

❷ Place one hand over the other, and press the acupoints on the back, along the Taiyang Bladder Meridian of Foot, as well as all the Jiaji points. Exert moderate pressure according to the patient's tolerance level.

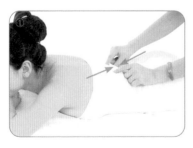

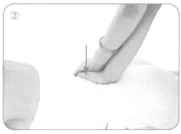

❸ Knead the sacroiliac joints on both sides of the patient's lumbosacral area repeatedly for 1 to 3 minutes. Massage the Baliao points one by one until the skin feels warm.

❹ Put the patient in the supine position, with their feet

together and knees bent. Hold the patient's ankle with both hands. Bend their knees close to their chest, and then make a circular movement.

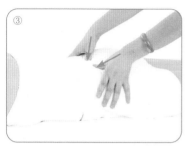 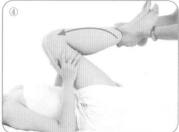

4. Other Methods for Lower Back Pain

Therapeutic treatment methods such as moxibustion, cupping, *gua sha* scraping, and exercise can be used alongside acupoint massage to alleviate lower back pain.

Moxibustion

When carrying out moxibustion therapy, it is important to note that the moxa stick should not contact the skin directly, to prevent burning. Measures must be taken to prevent the moxa ash from falling and igniting any combustible materials. During the treatment period, enhance the condition of your body through exercise and a healthy diet, and try to maintain a happy mood. Therapeutic treatment methods such as massage and cupping can be performed alongside moxibustion.

During an attack, moxibustion can be done once in the morning and once in the evening, with each session lasting 25 minutes. During the recovery period, carry out the treatment once a day for 15 minutes. For normal healthcare, do this twice a week, 10 minutes each time.

Moxibustion Points

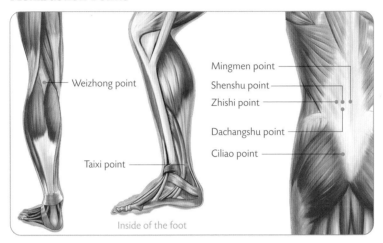

Mingmen point
Shenshu point
Zhishi point
Weizhong point
Dachangshu point
Ciliao point
Taixi point

Inside of the foot

Moxibustion Methods

❶ Ignite the moxa stick. Place it at about 1.5 to 3 cm away from the Shenshu point, and hold it there for 3 to 5 minutes.

❷ Ignite the moxa stick. Place it at about 1.5 to 3 cm away from the Ciliao point, and hold it there for 3 to 5 minutes.

❸ Ignite the moxa stick. Place it at about 1.5 to 3 cm away from the Weizhong point, and hold it there for 3 to 5 minutes.

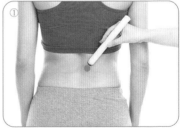

❹ Ignite the moxa stick. Place it at about 1.5 to 3 cm away from the Dachangshu point, and hold it there for 3 to 5 minutes.

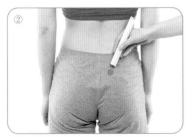

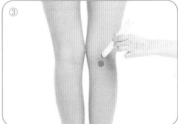

❺ Ignite the moxa stick. Place it at about 1.5 to 3 cm away from the Mingmen point, and hold it there for 3 to 5 minutes.

❻ Ignite the moxa stick. Place it at about 1.5 to 3 cm away from the Zhishi point, and hold it there for 3 to 5 minutes.

❼ Ignite the moxa stick. Place it at about 1.5 to 3 cm away from the Taixi point, and hold it there for 3 to 5 minutes.

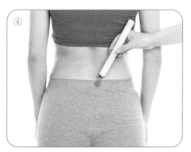
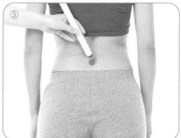
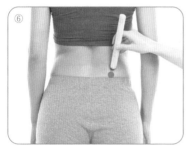
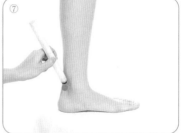

Cupping

Before a cupping session, have a simple back massage first, and then have the cups placed on the fleshier part of your body, either using the fire cupping or the air pump cups. Leave the cups on the affected spots, but not for too long. In your daily life, keep a regular routine and refrain from participating in strenuous exercise.

Cupping therapy should be done every other day during an attack period, and twice a week during the recovery period. For daily healthcare, cupping can be done once a week.

Cupping Points

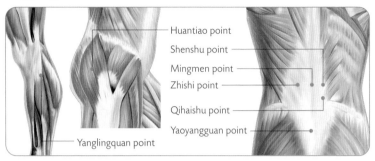

Huantiao point
Shenshu point
Mingmen point
Zhishi point
Qihaishu point
Yaoyangguan point
Yanglingquan point

Cupping Methods

❶ Put the cup on the Shenshu point for 5 to 10 minutes.

❷ Put the cup on the Qihaishu point for 5 to 10 minutes.

❸ Put the cup on the Huantiao point for 5 to 10 minutes.

❹ Put the cup on the Mingmen point for 5 to 10 minutes.

❺ Put the cup on the Zhishi point for 5 to 10 minutes.

❻ Put the cup on the Yaoyangguan point for 5 to 10 minutes.

❼ Put the cup on the Yanglingquan point for 5 to 10 minutes.

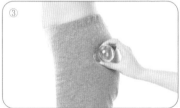

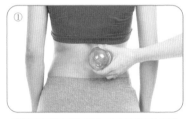

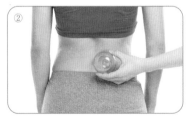

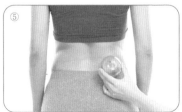

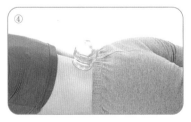

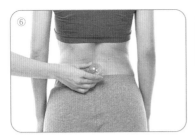
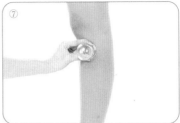

Gua Sha Scraping

After *gua sha* scraping, drink plenty of water and keep warm.
It is not advisable to take a bath immediately after a treatment.
Wait until the redness or red marks has disappeared before you
do scraping again. Take precautionary measures to avoid cold and
moisture. Maintain a daily routine, and do appropriate exercise.

Scraping therapy should be performed every other day in the
attack period, for 10 minutes each time. In the recovery period,
do it twice a week, for 5 minutes each time. For daily healthcare,
do it once a week, for 5 minutes each time.

Scraping Points

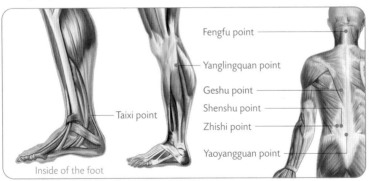

Fengfu point

Yanglingquan point

Geshu point

Shenshu point

Zhishi point

Yaoyangguan point

Taixi point

Inside of the foot

Scraping Methods

❶ Use the flat scraping method, increase the intensity, and
scrape the Geshu point repeatedly in an outward direction until

sha or red marks appear.

❷ Use the flat scraping method, increase the intensity, and scrape the Shenshu point repeatedly in an outward direction until red marks appear.

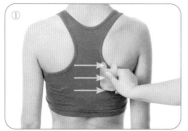
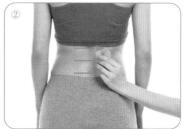

❸ Use the flat scraping method, increase the intensity, and scrape the Yaoyangguan point repeatedly in an outward direction until red marks appear.

❹ First press and knead the Fengfu point 5 to 10 times, and then scrape it repeatedly in a top-down direction until there is throbbing tenderness. The pressure exerted should not be too intense.

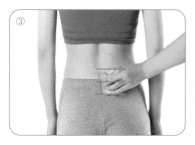
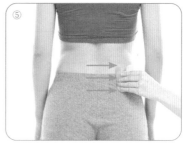

❺ Use the flat scraping method, increase the intensity, and scrape the Zhishi point repeatedly in an outward direction until red marks appear.

❻ Scrape the Taixi point, which is on the inner side

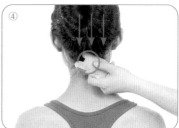

of the ankle. It is not advisable to use intense pressure on this point. Scrape repeatedly in a top-down direction until red marks appear on the skin surface and purple marks and lines begin to form under the skin.

❻ Use the flat scraping method on the Yanglingquan point, taking note that the pressure exerted on this point should not be intense. Scrape repeatedly in a top-down direction until the skin turns red on the surface and purple marks and lines begin to form under the skin.

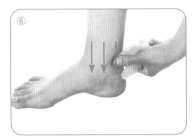 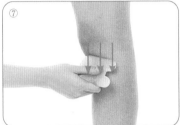

Exercise

Waist exercise should not be done immediately after a meal. When doing them, apply force evenly throughout. Keep your movements slow, avoid sudden starting and stopping, and perform the whole set of exercise for at least 15 minutes. Maintain a happy mood throughout.

During an attack period, exercise once a day for 30 minutes each time. In the recovery period, do it once every other day for 30 minutes each time. For daily healthcare, exercise twice a week for 20 minutes each time.

Exercise Methods

❶ Stand and raise your arms to form a horizontal line. Move them up and down, then left and right to exercise your lower back. When swinging your arms, remember to do corresponding movements at your waist as well.

❷ Move your upper body and lower body in opposite directions, that is, when your upper body moves to the left, your crotch region moves to the right, and vice versa.

❸ Mimic a boatman's rowing action with your arms, either forward or reverse. Keep the range of motion moderate, because if it is too large, it will be difficult to maintain balance, and if it is too small, the exercise will not have any effect.

❹ Hold your arms up horizontally. Use them to first drive the movement of your upper body, then your waist, rotating left and right. The whole action should be soothing, gentle, and relaxed, like willow leaves moving in the wind.

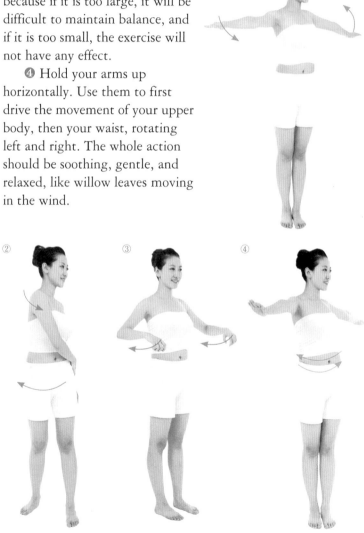

Chapter Five
Treatments to Relieve Leg Pain

The legs, needed for most sports, are the parts of our body that injure most easily. Rheumatoid arthritis, leg cramps, and Achilles tendon pain are some of the sequelae of poor care after leg injuries. Women tend to keep their legs exposed, even in cold weather, allowing Cold pathogens into the body. When they are young, they may not feel it. However, with time, this can become a hidden danger. Once the pain comes, it is difficult to get rid of, so looking after our legs should start early.

The knee joint is the most vulnerable part of the human body. It supports us when we stand, walk, run, and perform many movements. In recent years, knee joint pain has become a common ailment among young people who love sports. Once there is an injury in the knee joint, it is difficult to do any exercise or sports for length of time. This chapter offers guidance on how to avoid leg and knee pain.

1. Understanding Leg Pain

Issues such as external injuries, rheumatic arthritis, rheumatoid arthritis, gout, even heart disease, renal insufficiency, diabetes, osteoporosis, and other internal diseases are all possible causes of leg pain. Therefore, if you find yourself suffering, you should seek medical advice immediately.

Knowing about the Leg Joints
Our blood circulation is weakest in our legs and feet. When the downward flow of blood slows down, the speed of reflux will also decrease. For the blood to return to the heart, it has to go a long way. Therefore, great muscle strength is needed to return the

blood from the lower limbs to the heart.

Some people suffer weakness and heaviness in their legs and feet all year round. One of the reasons for this is that a large amount of blood is deposited in the lower limbs, and is not always able to flow back well. Another reason is that blood stasis in the legs increases the burden on the heart, and causes a gradual decrease in cardiac function.

When blood circulation in the lower limbs is improved, the legs and feet will get sufficient nutrition. The excretion ability of various metabolites will be enhanced, reducing the stimulation of the nerve ends, preventing spasm of the small blood vessels, and relieving pain. When blood in the lower limbs can flow back quickly, the pressure on the veins and localized swelling will be reduced.

Fundamental daily movements such as standing, walking, running, and jumping involve the movement of the knee joint. The knee joint's special meniscus is an axial pivot joint, and also has the characteristics of a ball and socket joint. It has a flexion and extension function, as well as a certain range of rotation.

According to modern anatomical research, the knee joint has a highly complex structure. A considerable number of ligaments and tendons are distributed around and inside it to ensure stability. This is because, although the surface area of the joint is large, it is in a shallow position and its joint capsule is thin and loose. The *Suwen* section of the *Huangdi Neijing* (known as the first book of TCM, composed of two sections, *Suwen* and *Lingshu*) refers to the knee as the "house of tendons." In the text, "knee" refers to the knee joint, and "tendon" refers to the muscles, tendons, ligaments, fascia, and other tissues. The "house of tendons" implies that the knee is the place where tendons converge.

As the largest, most complex, and most powerful joint in the human body, the knee bears almost all of the weight, and also undertakes the various movements of the legs. People who perform heavy physical labor or participate in vigorous jumping and strenuous exercise over long periods run a high risk of damaging their knee joints.

Causes of Leg Pain

There are many reasons for leg pain. If it becomes severe, you should seek medical attention. Speak with your doctor about the possible cause of your condition. The following are potential reasons for leg pain:

• Injury caused by sports or accidents: this can injure or damage the bones, joints, and ligaments.

• Prolonged periods of weight bearing and long-distance walking: this can cause strain and fatigue fractures in the muscles of the lower limbs.

• Diseases such as diabetes.

• Prolonged periods in a fixed posture or lifting heavy objects in the wrong way.

• Degenerative changes to the legs.

The invasion of Wind, Cold and Dampness pathogens can induce an attack of rheumatic arthritis, manifesting its uncomfortable symptoms such as swelling, numbness, heaviness, and weakness of knee and lower leg. Most of these symptoms occur on cold days, and are experienced mostly by middle-aged and elderly people, improving in warmer weather. Many image-conscious young people wear short skirts, thin trousers, and flimsy shoes, even in winter. While they may look good, this comes at the expense of their legs, which can become painful, and may develop rheumatic arthritis. People with rheumatic arthritis must keep warm, exercise, and take precautionary measures to prevent attacks. Rheumatic arthritis can also occur in summer, caused by the long-term use of air conditioning. In hot weather, the pores of our skin are open in order to dispel heat. Cold air from air-conditioning will gradually sink to the floor. Our knee joints and calves, as the lower limbs, will be the first to feel the cold. This cold air will gradually penetrate the tissues of the leg and knee.

The stability of the knee joint mainly depends on the ligaments and muscles, with the medial collateral ligaments as the most important. When the knee is slightly flexed, its stability is relatively poor. If it is subjected to a sudden external force that results in valgus[1] or varus[2], it may cause medial or lateral collateral ligament injury. The patient will experience severe knee pain. There will be swelling at the joint and surrounding it. Ecchymosis[3] will appear under the skin, there will be effusion in the joint, and activity will be limited, which will seriously affect the patient's work and life.

Some mountain climbers experience severe knee pain on the descent. Some elderly people suffer a bolt of pain when they stand up suddenly after sitting for a long time. Some people feel great pain when they walk up the stairs. The pain is often in the articular surface or the medial position of the patella. These symptoms manifest the same kind of problem, i.e., the softening and breaking down of the cartilage of the knee cap. The medical term for this is chondromalacia patella.

There are many ligaments surrounding the knee joint. The patella is actually located in front of the lower end of the femur when the knee is straightened. However, it will slide down along the thighbone when the knee is bent. The joint, composed of the patella and femur, is called the patellofemoral joint. When moving, the patella slides along a groove, and can easily shift slightly outside of it. Once the patella is displaced, it will cause a lot of pain.

There are two reasons why the patella can shift easily. One is that the soft tissue outside of it has stiffened. The other is that wear and tear has occurred between the patellofemoral joints. Therefore, strenuous exercise must be avoided, and traumatic impact should be inhibited, especially for the elderly.

Other causes of knee joint pain are:

• Meniscus injury: this is common among athletes.

---

[1] A deformity involving oblique displacement of part of a limb away from the midline.

[2] A deformity involving oblique displacement of part of a limb towards the midline.

[3] A discoloration of the skin resulting from bleeding underneath, typically caused by bruising.

• Strain on the fat pad of the knee: this is a condition that stems from external injury or long-term friction that causes congestion and hypertrophy resulting in inflammation of the fat pad.

• Hyperosteogeny: this is a degenerative change in the knee joint, consisting of wear and thinning of the articular cartilage.

Daily Care for Legs

Keeping warm. Muscles, tendons, ligaments, and fascia are characterized by their preference for warmth and dislike of cold. This is especially so in elderly people. Their ability to adjust and adapt to changes in environmental factors is weak. If they do not keep their lower limbs warm, vascular stenosis and sclerosis will worsen quickly. However, if they do, their symptoms will be reduced, and degradation of cartilage, vascular stenosis, and sclerosis can be prevented and alleviated.

Although excessive exercise and bone aging are common causes of knee pain, some pains are not caused by trauma. In many cases, cold is the cause of knee pain. People nowadays care a lot about external beauty. In winter, to avoid looking bloated in thick outfits, they neglect to wear warm clothes. They pay a high price—joint injury. Long-term cold can lead to muscular and vascular contraction, causing knee pain. Avoiding the cold and staying warm is vital in protecting the knee joint. At the same time, strengthening the leg muscles is also important. Wear knee pads in winter, and apply hot compresses to your knees regularly.

Hot compress. A simple home remedy for rheumatic arthritis is the salt compress. First, sew a book-sized pocket out of cotton fabric. Use double layer fabric, and line between the two layers with cotton or a material like sponge—neither too thick nor too thin. Put 1 kg of crude salt into a dry pan. Stir-fry it for several minutes. Turn off the heat when you hear popping sounds. Pour the salt into the bag and seal the opening of the pocket. Put the pocket on the painful area and cover it with a quilt. Do this for around one hour every night. It is a very effective treatment for rheumatic arthritis.

Self-massage. If swelling occurs with leg pain, a simple self-massage method can be used to relieve it. Sit on a chair with a 90° angle between your thighs and lower legs. Use your hollow fist to knock the whole thigh from top to bottom for 3 to 5 minutes. After applying this massage technique on the side of your thigh that faces outward, repeat it on the side that faces inward several times from top to bottom, to dredge the *qi* and blood.

Exercise. Young people who exercise often also suffer knee problems. People with joint pain or instability are more likely to fall, causing more serious damage to their joints. Exercise can enhance muscle strength, increase the strength and stability of the knee joints, and help control weight. Walking, swimming, water aerobics, and cycling are particularly effective forms of exercise. Rub the lower edge of the knee with both hands and fingers before exercising, to induce protective lubricant. Obesity is to be avoided. If you are obese, you must lose weight. Even a small amount of progress can make a big difference to your joints.

Cold compress. People who enjoy sport may suffer knee injuries due to long-term excessive exercise. In the case of an acute injury, a cold compress treatment can be used. Put ice water into a bag. Wrap the bag with a towel and place it on the affected area. Remove the bag after 20 to 30 minutes. Take a rest, and repeat the treatment when the skin temperature has returned to normal.

The right shoes. Wearing unsuitable shoes or walking long distances in slippers or high heels will subject the knee joint to long-term abnormal stress, resulting in chronic injury and pain. Some runners find that their knees become painful after a long session, but they are not able to pinpoint the reason. It could be time for them to change their running shoes. Wearing the right sports shoes is very important. It could also be due to an improper running posture, which should be adjusted quickly.

2. Common Acupoints for Relieving Leg Pain

When suffering a trauma, the pain can be unbearable, especially in the leg. Many people are afraid of aggravating the pain, so they try not to move too much. However, this is more likely to lead to varying degrees of adhesion and fibrosis of the muscles and ligaments at the site of the injury, intensifying the pain and extending the afflicted area. Perform massage therapy on the common acupoints for 30 minutes every day, for a cumulative effect. In addition, include 30 minutes of relaxation exercise every day, such as walking or *taiji*.

Knee pain is common among middle-aged and elderly people, as well as young people who do a lot of sport. Simple acupoint massage combined with other therapeutic TCM methods can alleviate pain and improve knee function. Knee pain can be relieved or cured if it receives timely medical treatment and proper care.

Twenty-Four Main Acupoints
Chengshan point: it has the function of relaxing the tendons and promoting blood circulation, and is one of the most commonly used points for the treatment of calf muscle spasm.

Chengjin point: it is located in the center of the gastrocnemius muscle. Pressing it can eliminate the spasm of this muscle and relieve pain in the calf.

Xuehai point: massage the Xuehai point with the tip of your thumb every morning and evening to treat knee pain and eczema.

Dubi point: located in the lateral depression of the patellar ligament, the Dubi point dredges meridians, activates collaterals, disperses Wind and Cold pathogens, regulates *qi*, relieves swelling and pain.

Kunlun point: located in the depression between the tip of the lateral ankle and the Achilles tendon. Massage this point every day to treat heel pain.

Liangqiu point: this point works well in the treatment

of acute knee joint diseases such as rheumatic arthritis, suprapatellar bursitis, and patella malacia.

Zusanli point: located on the lower limb, 3 cun below the Waixiyan point, the Zusanli point is one of the main points of the Yangming Stomach Meridian of Foot. It is a point that is commonly used for healthcare in TCM.

Weizhong point: with your thumb, press and knead the point located at the midpoint of the transverse crease of the popliteal fossa behind your knee cap. Do this every day to treat lower back and leg pain.

Yinlingquan point: hold the lower part of your knee with both hands, bend your thumbs, and knead the Yinlingquan point with the tips of your thumbs from bottom to top. This can alleviate knee pain.

Yanglingquan point: this point belongs to the gallbladder meridian[1]. It is an important point for the treatment of lower limb problems, such as knee pain.

Neixiyan point: this point is mainly used to treat arthritis and neuralgia of the knee, as well as numbness and motor system problems. The pressure on this point during massage should be light to avoid causing damage to the skin.

Feiyang point: this point can dredge the meridians at the back of the lower leg. For people suffering heaviness and pain in the lower leg, massage this point for the best effect.

Xiyangguan point: knead and press the Xiyangguan point with the pulp of your middle finger. You will feel throbbing

---

[1] The Shaoyang Gallbladder Meridian of Foot (GB) is one of the 12 meridians of the human body, along with the Taiyin Lung Meridian of Hand (LU), Jueyin Pericardium Meridian of Hand (PC), Shaoyin Heart Meridian of Hand (HT), Yangming Large Intestine Meridian of Hand (LI), Shaoyang *Sanjiao* Meridian of Hand (TE), Taiyang Small Intestine Meridian of Hand (SI), Yangming Stomach Meridian of Foot (ST), Taiyang Bladder Meridian of Foot (BL), Taiyin Spleen Meridian of Foot (SP), Jueyin Liver Meridian of Foot (LR), and Shaoyin Kidney Meridian of Foot (KI).

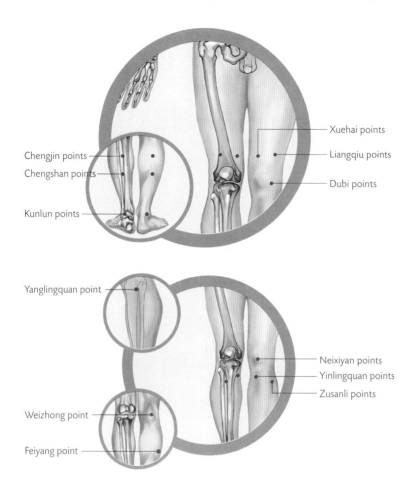

Xuehai points

Chengjin points

Liangqiu points

Chengshan points

Dubi points

Kunlun points

Yanglingquan point

Neixiyan points

Yinlingquan points

Zusanli points

Weizhong point

Feiyang point

pain. Massaging this point can improve swelling and pain in the knee joint.

Xiguan point: grasp and pinch the Xiguan point with the pulp of your thumb and index finger for 3 to 5 minutes to alleviate pain in the knee and lower limbs.

Chengfu point: massaging the Chengfu point with the pulp of your index finger, middle finger, and ring finger upward can alleviate lower back and leg pain, as well as lower limb paralysis.

Neixiyan point: the Xiyan points are located in the depression on both sides of the patellar ligament. The inner

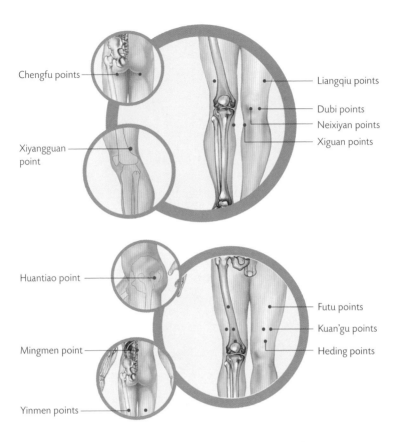

Chengfu points

Xiyangguan point

Liangqiu points

Dubi points

Neixiyan points

Xiguan points

Huantiao point

Mingmen point

Yinmen points

Futu points

Kuan'gu points

Heding points

point is called the Neixiyan (inner Xiyan) point. This point mainly treats arthritis and neuralgia of the knees, as well as numbness and motor system problems.

Dubi point: knee pain caused by strenuous exercise can be reduced by kneading the Dubi point for 5 minutes.

Liangqiu point: to treat arthritis of the knee, massage and nip-knead this point, which is located in the anterior femoral area.

Mingmen point: to treat cold limbs, massage the Mingmen point in the spine area for 3 minutes every day.

Yinmen point: applying moderate pressure, massage the Yinmen point with your hand or beat with a massage hammer or other massage tools. This can relax the tendons and collaterals, and strengthen the lower back and knee.

Futu point: using your fingers, knead and press the Futu point for about 3 minutes. This can alleviate lower back and knee pain as well as numbness of the lower limbs.

Huantiao point: kneading the Huantiao point often with the tip of your thumb with deep pressure can prevent lower limb paralysis and knee joint pain.

Kuan'gu point: kneading and pressing the Kuan'gu points with the pulp of your thumb for 1 to 3 minutes can strengthen the leg muscles and prevent leg problems.

Heding point: this point is located at the depression above the midpoint of the patellar base. Knead it often with the pulp of your fingers to treat knee joint pain.

3. Massage Methods for Legs

In addition to unsuitable exercise, strain, and cold, certain illnesses and disorders can lead to leg and knee pain. This section explains various causes of leg pain, and offers massage methods to alleviate it.

Knee Osteoarthritis

This is a condition that develops from degenerative pathological changes, which are usually related to overwork and trauma. When the patient feels unwell, it is not advisable to bend and extend the knee joint repeatedly nor press and knead the patella. On normal days, preventive measures must be taken to keep cold and moisture out. Do not stay in a fixed posture for too long, avoid fatigue, and relax your body. *Gua sha* scraping and moxibustion can be carried out to alleviate discomfort.

During an attack, massage should be performed once in the morning and once in the evening, with each session lasting 20 minutes. During the recovery period, massage once a day for 15 minutes. For normal healthcare, massage twice a week, for 15 minutes each time.

Massage Points

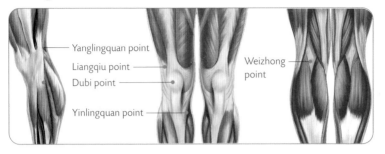

Yanglingquan point

Liangqiu point

Dubi point

Yinlingquan point

Weizhong point

Massage Methods

❶ Ask the patient to take the supine position. With four fingers and thumb, knead and pinch repeatedly for 5 to 10 minutes from the top of the patient's thigh to the lower part of their knee joint.

❷ With the patient still in the supine position, use the pulp of thumb, index finger, or middle finger, gently press the painful part of the knee joint. Then, press in turn the Liangqiu, Weizhong, Dubi, Yinlingquan, and Yanglingquan points for 1 to 3 minutes respectively.

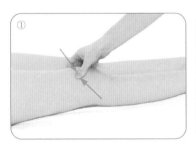

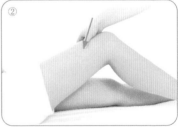

❸ Put the patient in the prone position. First, press the sore part of the knee joint with the pulp of thumb or other fingers. Next, knead and pinch the calf for several minutes, and then rotate gently to move the knee joint.

❹ If the swelling on the knee is obvious, after the above manipulation, use the first third of the thumb pulp to nip-knead the swollen area, with as much pressure as the patient can tolerate. Because the stimulation from the nip-knead technique is intense, after performing this manipulation, you can gently knead the local area for several minutes to soothe any pain.

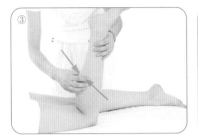 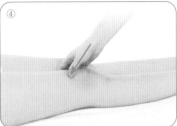

Chondromalacia Patella

Patella malacia is a result of a disorder of the biomechanical relationship in the patella joint, which is usually related to natural wear and tear. Taking care of your knee joint should begin as early as possible. Patients should avoid strenuous exercise, maintain a reasonable weight, keep warm, and perform massage every day.

During an attack, massage should be performed once in the morning and once in the evening, with each session lasting 20 minutes. During the recovery period, massage once a day for 15 minutes. For normal healthcare, massage twice a week, for 15 minutes each time.

Massage Points

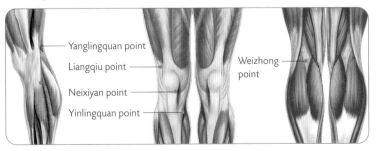

Yanglingquan point

Liangqiu point

Neixiyan point

Yinlingquan point

Weizhong point

Massage Methods

❶ Put the patient in the supine position with their knee flexed. Use the pulp of thumb to press and knead the Liangqiu, Neixiyan, Weizhong, Yinlingquan, and Yanglingquan points around the knee joint, for about 30 seconds each.

❷ With the patient still in the supine position, massage him/her using the rolling technique for 2 minutes from one-third below the thigh to one-third above the calf. Then, put the patient in the prone position. Cushion their calf with a pillow, and then use the same massage technique on the back of their knee joint and surrounding area for 2 minutes.

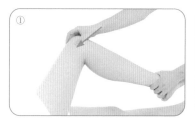
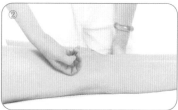

❸ With the patient in the supine position, use the hypothenar of the palm to press and knead both sides of the patella repeatedly. Then, tap the upper and lower edges of the patella with the tips of your middle three fingers for a few minutes. After that, press and release the patella with your palm 3 to 5 times.

❹ With the patient still in the supine position, pinch the area around the patella with the tips of five fingers. Next, rub up and down toward their thigh and calf with deep pressure. Finally, hold the patient's ankle with one hand and press the patella with the other hand, and perform the extension and flexion movement of the knee joint 3 to 5 times.

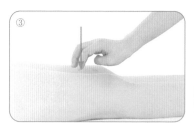
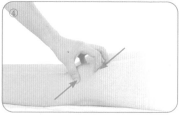

Rheumatic Arthritis of the Knee

Rheumatic arthritis of the knee is one of the main manifestations of rheumatic fever. It usually starts with acute fever and joint pain. Patients should keep warm, avoid cold and humidity, take more exercise, have a balanced diet, and boost immunity. Avoid climbing mountains and going up and down the stairs.

During an attack, massage should be performed once in the morning and once in the evening, with each session lasting 20 minutes. During the recovery period, massage once a day for 15 minutes. For normal healthcare, massage three times a week, for 15 minutes each time.

Massage Points

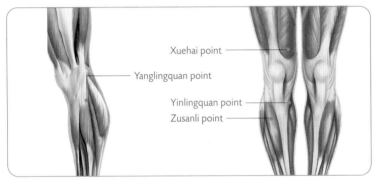

Xuehai point

Yanglingquan point

Yinlingquan point
Zusanli point

Massage Methods

❶ Put the patient in the supine position and stand next to him/her. Press their patella tightly with palm, rubbing in a circular movement in one direction, either leftward or rightward, gradually increasing the pressure. Repeat this action for 2 to 3 minutes.

❷ Use thumb and the other four fingers of either one hand or both hands to nip-pinch with pressure on the affected quadriceps femoris (the muscle at the anterior compartment of the thigh). Nip-pinch 5 to 6 times from the knee to the end of the thigh, gradually increasing the pressure.

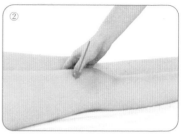

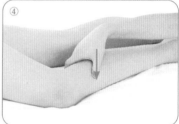

❸ Press the tender points around the knee with thumb and index finger, and increase the pressure from light to heavy, then from heavy to light for about 1 minute.

❹ Press the patient's Xuehai, Yinlingquan, Yanglingquan, and Zusanli points with thumb, with moderate pressure, for 1 minute each.

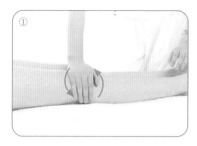

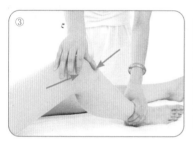

Leg Cramps

Leg cramps occur mainly in the muscles of the calves and toes, and are usually related to excessive fatigue. Patients must remember to rest, keep warm, and avoid subjecting the leg muscles to cold. Make sure you get enough sleep, and take a calcium supplement.

During an attack, massage should be performed once in the morning and once in the evening, with each session lasting 20 minutes. During the recovery period, massage once a day for 15 minutes. For normal healthcare, massage 3 times a week, for 15 minutes each time.

Massage Points

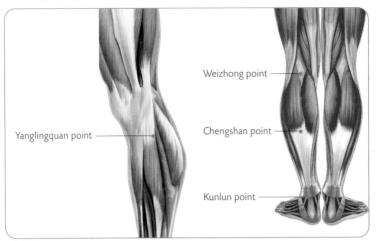

Weizhong point

Yanglingquan point

Chengshan point

Kunlun point

Massage Methods

❶ Put the patient in the prone position. Using thumb and the other four fingers, grasp and pinch the patient's calf muscles for 1 minute to relax them. Then, press with deep pressure on the cramped muscle to calm the nerves and relieve pain.

❷ Put the patient in the prone position. First, put the tip of thumb on the popliteal fossa behind the patient's knee joint, put other four fingers on the outside of the knee, and rub the Weizhong point with deep pressure for 1 minute. Then, with deep pressure, press and knead the Yanglingquan point for 1 minute with the pulp of your thumb on the outer side of the affected calf, with the other four fingers on the muscle belly of the lower limb.

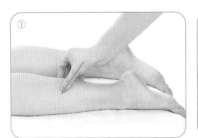

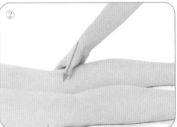

❸ With the patient still in the prone position, use the tip of thumb to pinch and press the Chengshan point for 1 minute. Then, press the Chengshan and Kunlun points for 1 minute respectively with the pulp of thumb or middle finger.

❹ During an episode of leg cramps, the patient should sit up instead of lying down, and stretch the affected leg. Then, the patient uses his/her own thumb to press and knead the calf muscles with deep pressure from the popliteal fossa to the Achilles tendon for several minutes until the calf muscles relax.

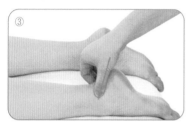
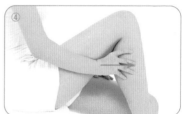

Heel Pain

Heel pain is aggravated by walking. It is usually related to a deficiency in kidney *yang*[1]. People with this condition should nourish their kidneys to strengthen *yang*, and reduce local compression. Thin-soled cloth shoes should be avoided. Pedal your feet frequently. Treatments include local physiotherapy and hot compress. Moxibustion and cupping can also be carried out to alleviate discomfort.

During an attack, massage should be performed once in the morning and once in the evening, with each session lasting 20 minutes. During the recovery period, massage once a day for 15 minutes. For normal healthcare, massage twice a week, for 15 minutes each time.

---

[1] Kidney *yang* (the *yang qi* of the kidney, as opposed to kidney *yin*) is the kidney system's function of warmth, drive, motion, vitality, and *qi* transformation.

Massage Points

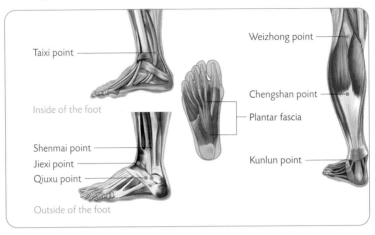

Taixi point

Inside of the foot

Weizhong point

Chengshan point

Plantar fascia

Shenmai point
Jiexi point
Qiuxu point

Kunlun point

Outside of the foot

Massage Methods

❶ Get the patient to lie prone and relax their whole body. Stand behind him/her. First, use the pulp of thumb to grasp and pinch and press and knead several times, from top to bottom from the gastrocnemius muscle of the patient's calf to the calcaneus. Then, press the Weizhong, Chengshan, Kunlun, Shenmai, Qiuxu, Jiexi, and Taixi points.

❷ With the patient still in the prone position, first use the pulp of thumbs to follow the plantar fascia[1] from the heel to the toe. Rub and knead several times to make it hot. Then, with the

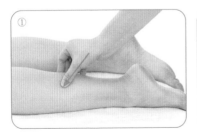

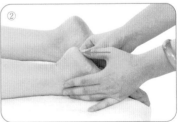

---

[1] The plantar fascia covers the plantar structure, which is the aponeurosis located in the deep subcutaneous tissue of the plantar.

tip of your finger, gently pluck in a perpendicular direction on the plantar fascia several times.

❸ With the patient in the supine position, flex the affected side of the knee joint with the sole facing upward. First, press the patient's heel and its surrounding parts repeatedly. Then, overlap the pulp of both thumbs and press the heel successively from back to front, from the outer side to inner side for 1 minute, with slightly more pressure.

❹ Get the patient to lie on their back. Stand at the end of the bed. First, hold the heel of the affected side with both hands, and pull-stretch and rotate the ankle several times; then, ask the patient to move their ankle several times.

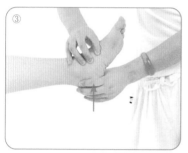
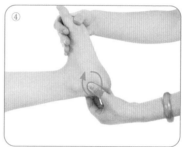

Knee Bursitis

Knee bursitis around the knee joint is commonly seen in repeated, long-term, and continual rubbing and compressing of the joint, which is related to excessive local wear. Patients should apply a cold compress, take enough rest, and exercise with the right posture. Manage your body weight and coordinate the movements of your knee joints carefully.

During an attack, massage should be performed once in the morning and once in the evening, with each session lasting 10 minutes. During the recovery period, massage once a day for 10 minutes. For normal healthcare, massage twice a week, for 10 minutes each time.

Massage Points

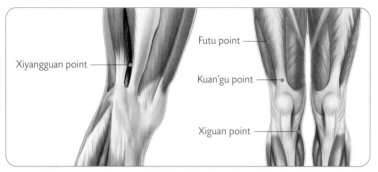

Massage Methods

❶ Locate the Xiyangguan point on the outer side of the knee joint; knead and press this point with the pulp of your thumb. When the patient begins to feel a throbbing pain, rest for a few seconds before continuing the manipulation. Pressing this point regularly can improve and treat knee swelling and pain.

❷ The Futu points are located in the thick muscles in the anterior of the thighs. The best way to knead them is to use pressing manipulation with kneading, pressing each point for about 3 minutes, and resting for a few seconds in between. Regular pressing can relieve lower back and knee pain, and numbness of the lower limbs.

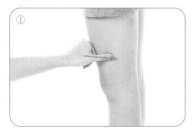
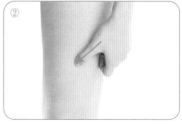

❸ The Xiguan point is close to the knee joint. Press it with the pulp of the thumb for 3 to 5 minutes, then rest for a few seconds. Pressing this point regularly can relieve knee pain.

❹ Each of the Kuan'gu points is located at 1.5 cun respectively on the left and right of the Liangqiu point, 2 cun on the outer side of the bottom of the patella. Regularly kneading the Kuan'gu point with the pulp of the thumb for 1 to 3 minutes each time can strengthen the leg muscles and alleviate bursitis around the knee joint.

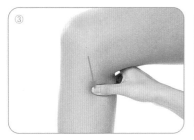 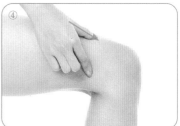

Synovial Plica Syndrome

This commonly occurs when the knee is subjected to direct trauma or chronic strain. It is usually related to inflammatory hyperemia and edema caused by external stimuli. Patients should rest well and avoid strenuous exercise.

During an attack, massage should be performed once in the morning and once in the evening, with each session lasting 20 minutes. During the recovery period, massage twice a day for 20 minutes. For normal healthcare, massage once on alternate days, for 20 minutes each time.

Massage Points

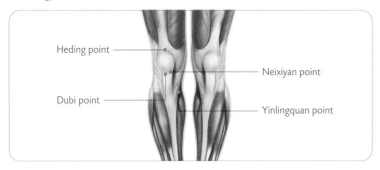

Heding point

Neixiyan point

Dubi point

Yinlingquan point

Massage Methods

❶ Knead and press the Heding point with the pulp of thumb regularly, 3 times a day, 150 times each time. This manipulation can treat both knee pain and limited flexion and extension.

❷ Pressing the Neixiyan point regularly with the pulp of the thumb can be effective in the treatment of knee hyperplasia and fibrosis. Apply light pressure to avoid damaging the skin. Carry out this manipulation for both the right and left side, 3 times a day, 150 times each time.

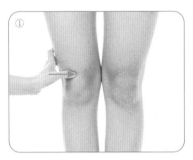
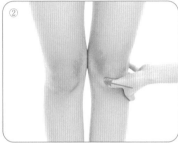

❸ Pressing and kneading the Yinlingquan point with the pulp of the thumb 200 times can alleviate pain in the abdomen and knees.

❹ Kneading and pressing the Dubi point for 5 minutes can reduce knee pain caused by strenuous exercise. Massaging the Dubi points with the pulp of the index finger persistently over time, each time for 1 to 3 minutes can improve conditions such as knee pain and weakness.

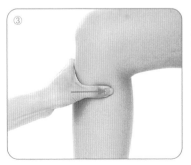
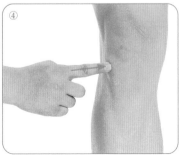

4. Other Methods for Leg Pain

In addition to acupoint massage, you can also use moxibustion, cupping, *gua sha* scraping, food therapy, and exercise to alleviate leg pain. These methods are easy to manage and can be carried out anytime, anywhere.

Moxibustion

Moxibustion sessions should not be too long, especially if it is your first time. It is not advisable to carry out this treatment when you are extremely tired, nor when you are dizzy. Immediately after moxibustion, avoid using cold water and taking a bath. Instead, drink warm water and keep warm.

During an attack, moxibustion can be done once a day, with each session lasting 5 minutes. During the recovery period, carry out the treatment once on alternate days, each time for 5 minutes. For normal healthcare, do this twice a week, for 5 minutes each time.

Moxibustion Points

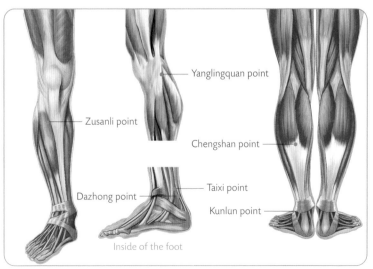

Yanglingquan point

Zusanli point

Chengshan point

Taixi point

Dazhong point

Kunlun point

Inside of the foot

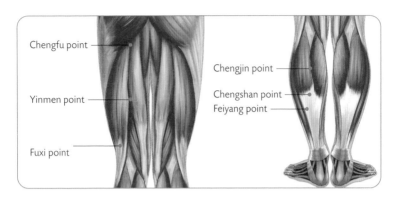

Chengfu point

Yinmen point

Fuxi point

Chengjin point

Chengshan point
Feiyang point

Moxibustion Methods

Leg Pain

❶ Ignite the moxa stick. Place it 1.5 to 3 cm away from the Chengshan point, and hold it there for 3 to 5 minutes.

❷ Ignite the moxa stick. Place it 1.5 to 3 cm away from the Zusanli point, and hold it there for 3 to 5 minutes.

❸ Ignite the moxa stick. Place it 1.5 to 3 cm away from the Yanglingquan point, and hold it there for 3 to 5 minutes.

❹ Ignite the moxa stick. Place it 1.5 to 3 cm away from the Taixi point, and hold it there for 3 to 5 minutes.

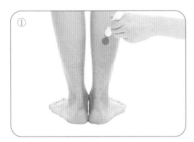

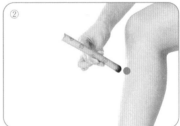

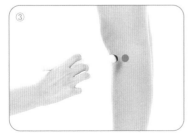

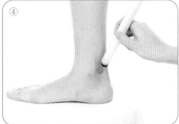

❺ Ignite the moxa stick. Place it 1.5 to 3 cm away from the Dazhong point, and hold it there for 3 to 5 minutes.

❻ Ignite the moxa stick. Place it 1.5 to 3 cm away from the Kunlun point, and hold it there for 3 to 5 minutes.

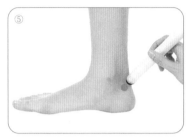

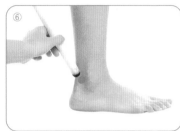

Knee Pain

❶ Ignite the moxa stick. Place it 1.5 to 3 cm away from the Chengfu point, and hold it there for 3 to 5 minutes.

❷ Ignite the moxa stick. Place it 1.5 to 3 cm away from the Yinmen point, and hold it there for 3 to 5 minutes.

❸ Ignite the moxa stick. Place it 1.5 to 3 cm away from the Fuxi point, and hold it there for 3 to 5 minutes.

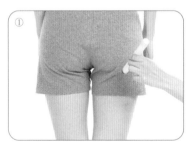

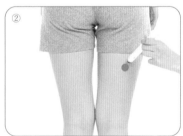

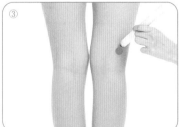

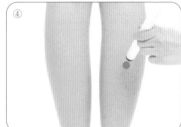

❹ Ignite the moxa stick. Place it 1.5 to 3 cm away from the Chengjin point, and hold it there for 3 to 5 minutes.

❺ Ignite the moxa stick. Place it 1.5 to 3 cm away from the Chengshan point, and hold it there for 3 to 5 minutes.

❻ Ignite the moxa stick. Place it 1.5 to 3 cm away from the Feiyang point, and hold it there for 3 to 5 minutes.

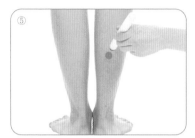
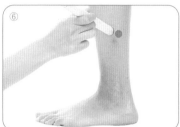

Cupping

It is not advisable to have cupping therapy when you are too full or hungry. You can use either the fire cupping or air pump cups. Have a simple massage first. Do not leave the cups on for too long each time. After a cupping session, keep warm; refrain from taking a bath immediately, and avoid the wind. Avoid being in humid environments for a long period of time. Cupping can be combined with *gua sha* scraping and massage therapy.

Cupping therapy is to be done once every other day during the attack period, each time for 10 minutes. During the recovery period, do it twice a week, each time for 10 minutes. For daily healthcare, cupping can be done once a week, for 10 minutes each time.

Cupping Methods

Leg Pain

❶ Put the cup on the Chengfu point for 5 to 10 minutes.

❷ Put the cup on the Yinmen point for 5 to 10 minutes.

❸ Put the cup on the Huantiao point for 5 to 10 minutes.

❹ Put the cup on the Feiyang point for 5 to 10 minutes.

❺ Put the cup on the Yanglingquan point for 5 to 10 minutes.

❻ Put the cup on the Chengshan point for 5 to 10 minutes.

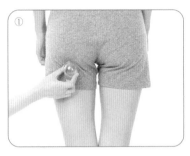

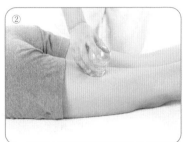

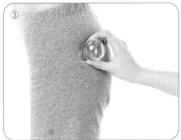

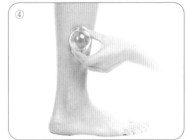

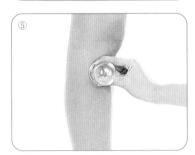

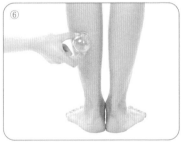

Knee Pain

❶ Put the cup on the Fuxi point for 5 to 10 minutes.

❷ Put the cup on the Chengjin point for 5 to 10 minutes.

❸ Put the cup on the Yanglingquan point for 5 to 10 minutes.

❹ Put the cup on the Xuehai point for 5 to 10 minutes.

❺ Put the cup on the Liangqiu point for 5 to 10 minutes.

❻ Put the cup on the Zusanli point for 5 to 10 minutes.

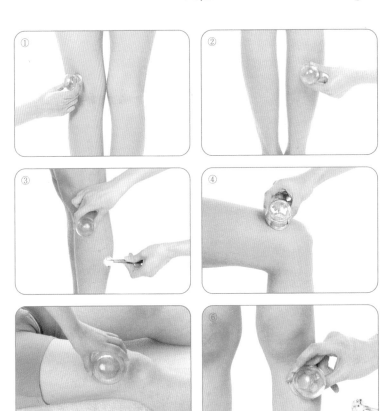

Cupping Points

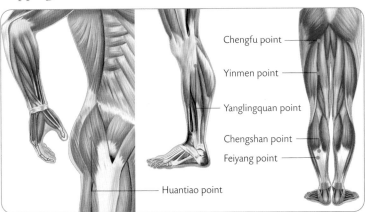

Chengfu point

Yinmen point

Yanglingquan point

Chengshan point

Feiyang point

Huantiao point

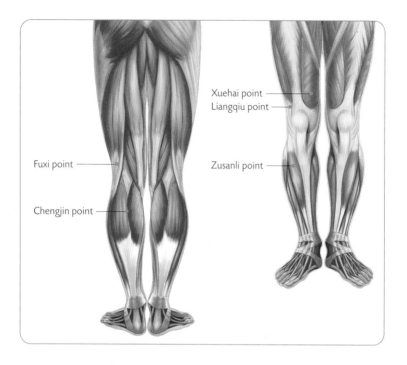

Gua Sha Scraping

People who are underweight should not undergo scraping therapy. Each session should not exceed 20 minutes. Remember to disinfect the scraping board before using it. A simple massage can be carried out before a scraping session. The pressure applied should not be too heavy, and it is not advisable to scrape one place repeatedly. Avoid taking a bath immediately after a treatment, but drink some water. Stay away from wind, and dress warmly. Exercise regularly, and eat a light daily diet.

Scraping therapy is to be performed twice weekly in the attack period, for 10 minutes each time. In the recovery period, do it once a week, for 10 minutes each time. For daily healthcare, do it twice every 3 weeks, for 10 minutes each time.

Scraping Points

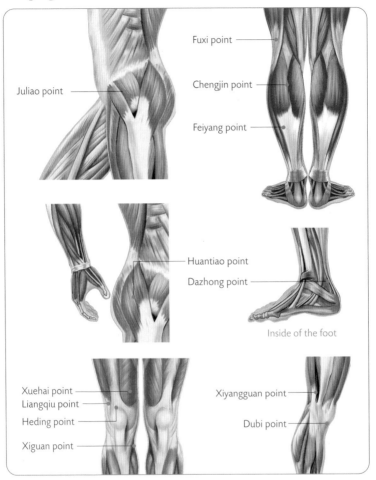

Fuxi point

Chengjin point

Feiyang point

Juliao point

Huantiao point

Dazhong point

Inside of the foot

Xuehai point
Liangqiu point
Heding point
Xiguan point

Xiyangguan point

Dubi point

Scraping Methods

Leg Pain

❶ Use the flat scraping method, increase the intensity, and scrape the Dazhong point in an outward direction repeatedly until *sha* or red marks appear.

❷ Use the flat scraping method, increase the intensity, and scrape the Chengjin point in a top-down direction repeatedly until red marks appear.

❸ Use the flat scraping method, increase the intensity, and scrape the Juliao point in an outward direction repeatedly until red marks appear.

❹ First press and knead the Fuxi point 5 to 10 times, and then scrape this point in an outward direction repeatedly with a scraping board until there is throbbing tenderness. Note: the pressure applied should not be too heavy.

❺ Use the flat scraping method, increase the intensity, and scrape the Feiyang point from top-down direction, repeatedly until or red marks appear.

❻ Use the flat scraping method, increase the intensity, and scrape the Huantiao point in an outward direction, repeatedly until red marks appear.

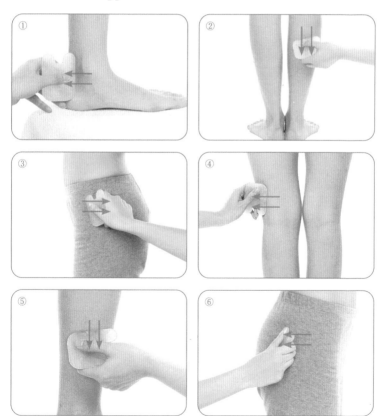

Knee Pain

❶ Use the flat scraping method, increase the intensity, and scrape the Dubi point from top-down direction, repeatedly until red marks appear.

❷ Use the flat scraping method, increase the intensity, and scrape the Heding point from top-down direction, repeatedly until red marks appear.

❸ Use the flat scraping method, increase the intensity, and scrape the Xiyangguan point from top-down direction, repeatedly until red marks appear.

❹ First, press and knead the Xiguan point 5 to 10 times. Next, use the scraping board to scrape this point back and forth from the top down until there is throbbing tenderness. Note: the pressure applied should not be too heavy.

❺ Use the flat scraping method, increase the intensity, and scrape the Xuehai point in an outward direction repeatedly until red marks appear.

❻ Use the flat scraping method, increase the intensity, and scrape the Liangqiu point in a top-down direction repeatedly until red marks appear.

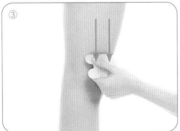

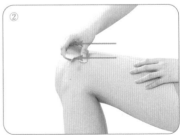

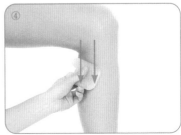

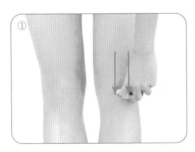

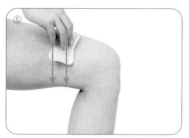

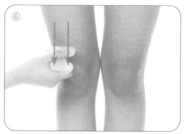

Exercise

The movements in leg and knee exercise should be uniform and slow; avoid starting suddenly and stopping abruptly. The whole set of movements should be carried out for at least 15 minutes, and the number of times should be based on an individual's tolerance level. It is important to keep hydrated and change out of wet, sweaty clothes. Swimming is a good form of exercise for knee pain. Hot compress treatment can also be carried out.

Exercise Methods

Leg Pain

❶ Stand naturally, supporting yourself with one hand on the wall. Point the tip of one foot forward and upward, then swing it backwards forcefully, straightening the back of the foot. Do this with the other leg. Repeat for both legs for 3 to 5 minutes.

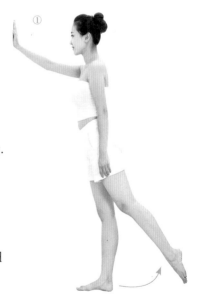

❷ First, put one leg on the bed, table, or stool, and beat it gently. Then slowly straighten the lower limbs and try to bend your head towards your foot. Repeat with the other leg.

Do this exercise interchangeably between the two legs for 3 to 5 minutes.

❸ Put your feet together side by side. Bend your knees slightly, and put your hands on your knees. Twist your knees clockwise and counterclockwise for 5 minutes respectively.

❹ Stretch out your hands and keep them parallel. Look forwards, suck in your stomach, and hold your breath. Then, bend your knees, keep them slightly apart, and with your feet pointing outward, breathe and squat down and stand up. Do this up-down exercise repeatedly for 5 minutes.

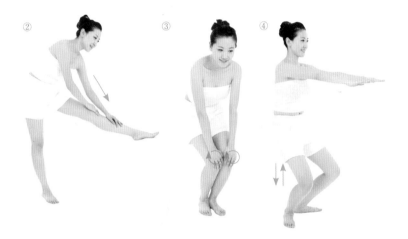

Knee Pain

❶ To avoid injury, it is important to warm up before exercise. Simply stretch every part of your body or walk for a few minutes.

❷ People with poor knee joints can start with simple movements. Lie flat. Bend one leg and step on the ground. Straighten the other leg and lift it up to the level of the knee joint of the bent leg and hold it there for 3 seconds. Alternate the two legs and do 3 sets, 10 times for each set.

❸ Stand facing the back of the chair, and hold it with your hands. Lift one foot backwards, as high as you can. Hold it there for 3 seconds. Do the same with the other leg. Do 3 sets of this every day, each set for 15 minutes. If you find this action too easy, you can add weight to your ankle, such as a bottle of mineral water, and increase the weight gradually.

❹ Lie in the prone position. Tighten the muscles of the hips, thighs, and behind the calves. Lift both your legs together and keep them there for 3 to 5 seconds. Lower them and repeat. Do this 10 to 15 times then rest. You can also add weight to your ankle. This action should not cause lower back pain. If it does, stop exercising immediately.

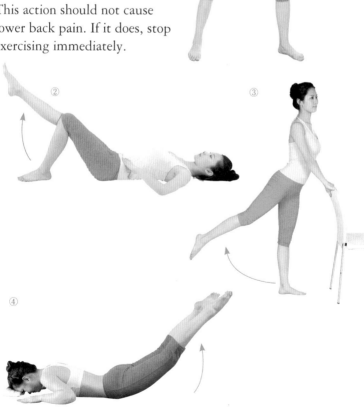

Food Therapy

Keep your tableware clean. Exercise appropriately, and avoid overeating. Do not eat overnight leftovers. Take note of the shelf life of your food, and choose ingredients that are in season.

Recipes

❶ Lychee, Lotus Seeds, and Chinese Yam Stew

Ingredients: 100 g each of lychees with the seeds removed, lotus seeds, Chinese yam.

Method: wash the lychees and lotus seeds. Wash and peel the Chinese yam before cutting it into pieces. Put them in a bowl, add a suitable amount of water, and cook.

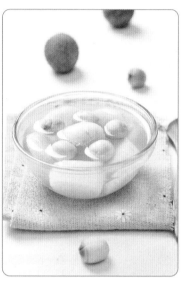

Function: tonifies *qi* and blood, nourishes the muscles and veins.

Note: lychees should not be eaten in large quantities.

❷ Black Bean Porridge

Ingredients: 20 g black beans, 60 g round-grained rice, brown sugar and sesame seeds to taste.

Method: wash the round-grained rice. Soak the black beans in warm water for one night, then wash. Boil both the rice and beans in a pot for a few minutes. Add the brown sugar and sesame seeds and continue cooking until the rice becomes

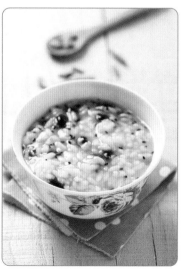

a thick, sticky porridge.

Function: dispels Wind pathogen, promotes blood circulation, induces diuresis, and reduces swelling.

❸ Stir-Fried Shrimp and Chives

Ingredients: 150 g chives, 250 g shelled shrimp, salt to taste.

Method: wash the chives and cut them into short strips. Wash the shelled shrimp. Heat oil in the pan and fry the shrimp until they turn red. Add the chives and stir fry until cooked. Add salt to taste.

Function: tonifies the kidneys and strengthens the bones.

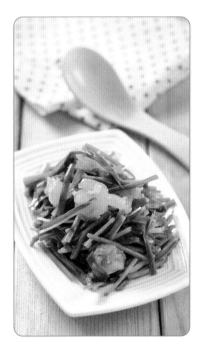

Appendix

Location of Acupoints

Acupoint	Code	Location	Fast Localization
Bailao	BL 31–34	There are eight Baliao points in total, four on each side of the sacral spine. These are the upper, secondary, middle and lower Baliao points. They are located respectively in the first, second, third and fourth posterior sacral foramina (opening between vertebrae).	Refer to the location.
Baihui	GV 20	On the head, 5 cun superior to the anterior hairline, on the anterior midline.	When seated, in the depression at the crossing point of the arch connecting the ear apex and the midline on the head.
Bi'nao	LI 14	On the lateral aspect of the arm on both sides of the body, just anterior to the border of the deltoid muscle, 7 cun superior to Quchi point (LI 11).	With elbow flexed and the deltoid muscle bulged while forming a fist, the point is on the inferior portion of the deltoid of the medial side, feeling soreness and distention on palpation.

Acupoint	Code	Location	Fast Localization
Chengfu	BL 36	On both sides of the buttock region, at the midpoint of the gluteal crease.	In prone, at the midpoint of gluteal transverse crease, feeling soreness and distention on palpation.
Chengjin	BL 56	On the posterior aspect of both legs, between the two muscle bellies of the gastrocnemius muscle, 5 cun distal to the popliteal crease.	In prone, in the center on the top of muscle of the leg in fully contraction, feeling soreness and distention on pressure.
Chengshan	BL 57	On the posterior aspect of both legs, at the connecting point of the calcaneal tendon with the two muscle bellies of the gastrocnemius muscle.	In prone, the midpoint between the center of the popliteal crease and the tip of the external malleolus.
Chize	LU 5	On the anterior aspect of the elbow, at the cubital crease, in the depression lateral to the biceps brachii tendon.	Elbow flexed, on the lateral border of the tendon.
Ciliao	BL 32	On both sides of sacral region, in the second posterior sacral foramen.	Refer to the location.

Acupoint	Code	Location	Fast Localization
Dachangshu	BL 25	On both sides of lumbar region, at the same level as the inferior border of the spinous process of the fourth lumbar vertebra, 1.5 cun lateral to the posterior midline.	Refer to the location.
Daling	PC 7	On the anterior aspect of both wrists, between the tendons of palmaris longus and the flexor carpi radialis, on the palmar wrist crease.	Wrist flexed slightly and fist made, the midpoint of the first transverse crease of wrist and between two tendons.
Dazhu	BL 11	On both sides of upper back region, at the same level as the inferior border of the spinous process of the first thoracic vertebra, 1.5 cun lateral to the posterior midline.	Neck flexed, 1.5 cun breadth lateral to the lower border of that one more vertebra down from the top vertebra.
Dazhong	KI 4	On the medial aspect of both feet, posteroinferior to the medial malleolus, superior to the calcaneus, in the depression anterior to medial attachment of the calcaneal tendon.	In sitting or supine, at the level of the inferior border of the medial malleolus, anterior to the Achilles tendon.

Acupoint	Code	Location	Fast Localization
Dazhui	GV 14	In the posterior region of the neck, in the depression inferior to the spinous process of the seventh cervical vertebra, on the posterior midline.	With head lowered, in the depression of the lower border of the biggest vertebra of the neck.
Dubi	ST 35	On the anterior aspect of both knees, in the depression lateral to the patellar ligament.	In a sitting position, extending the lower limbs forcefully and straightly, in the depression on the inferior lateral border of the knee.
Ermen	TE 21	On both sides of the face, in the depression between the supratragic notch and the condylar process of the mandible.	Anterior to the upper border of the tragus, in the depression when the mouth is open.
Feiyang	BL 58	On the posterolateral aspect of both legs, between the inferior border of the lateral head of the gastrocnemius muscle and the calcaneal tendon, at the same level as 7 cun proximal to Kunlun point (BL 60).	1 cun lateral and inferior to Chengshan point (BL 57).

Acupoint	Code	Location	Fast Localization
Fengchi	GB 20	In the posterior region of both sides of the neck, inferior to the occipital bone, in the depression between the origins of sternocleidomastoid and the trapezius muscles.	In a sitting position, in the depression on the lateral border of the two tendons on the back of head, at the level of earlobe.
Fengfu	GV 16	In the posterior region of the neck, directly inferior to the external occipital protuberance, in the depression between the trapezius muscle.	1 cun within the posterior hairline, along the spine.
Fengmen	BL 12	On both sides of upper back region, at the same level as the inferior border of the spinous process of the second thoracic vertebra, 1.5 cun lateral to the posterior midline.	Neck flexed, 1.5 cun lateral to the lower border of two more vertebras down from the most outstanding vertebra.
Futu	ST 32	On the anterolateral aspect of both thighs, on the line connecting the lateral end of the base of the patella with the anterior superior iliac spine, 6 cun superior to the base of the patella.	Flex the knees 90°, cup the hand on the knee, place the midpoint of the 1st transverse crease of the palm to the midpoint on the upper border of the patella, the point is where the tip of middle finger touches.

Acupoint	Code	Location	Fast Localization
Fuxi	BL 38	On the posterior aspect of both knees, just medial to the biceps femoris tendon, 1 cun proximal to the popliteal crease.	Refer to the location.
Geshu	BL 17	On both sides of upper back region, at the same level as the inferior border of the spinous process of the seventh thoracic vertebra, 1.5 cun lateral to the posterior midline.	1.5 cun lateral to the lower border of the vertebra at the level of the inferior scapular angle.
Hegu	LI 4	On the dorsum of both hands, radial to the midpoint of the second metacarpal bone.	Closing the index finger and thumb, on the top of the muscle.
Heding	EX-LE 2	In front of both knees, at the depression on the top of the center point of the patellar bottom.	On the knee, in the depression of the center on the upper border of the patella.
Houxi	SI 3	On the dorsum of both hands, in the depression proximal to the ulnar side of the fifth metacarpophalangeal joint, at the border between the red and white flesh.	Forming a fist, on the posterior border of the fifth metacarpophalangeal joint, at the border between the red and white flesh.

Acupoint	Code	Location	Fast Localization
Huantiao	GB 30	On both sides of the buttock region, at the junction of the lateral one-third and medial two-thirds of the line connecting the prominence of the great trochanter with sacral hiatus.	Lying on one side, the upper leg flexed, matching the thumb transverse crease with the greater trochanter, the thumb pointing the spine, in the depression where the thumb tip touches.
Jiaji	EX-B 2	On the spine area, both sides of the spinous from the first thoracic to the fifth lumbar, 0.5 cun lateral to the middle line of back, there are seventeen points each side.	0.5 cun lateral to each vertebra from the top vertebra at the junction of neck and back.
Jianjing	GB 21	At the midpoint of the line connecting the spinous process of the seventh cervical vertebra with the lateral end of both acromia.	Refer to the location.
Jianliao	TE 14	On both shoulder girdles, in the depression between the acromial angle and the greater tubercle of the humerus.	Refer to the location.

Acupoint	Code	Location	Fast Localization
Jianyu	LI 15	On both shoulder girdles, in the depression between the anterior end of the lateral border of the acromion and the greater tubercle of the humerus.	Seated straight, flex the elbow and raise the arm as high as the shoulder. The point is in the depression present on the shoulder when the middle finger presses the shoulder tip.
Jianzhen	SI 9	On both shoulder girdles, posteroinferior to the shoulder joint, 1 cun superior to the posterior axillary fold.	In a sitting position with shoulder relaxed, 1 cun above the end of the posterior axillary fold.
Jianzhongshu	SI 15	On both sides of the upper back region, at the same level as the inferior border of the spinous process of the seventh cervical vertebra, 2 cun lateral to the posterior midline.	Lowering the head, 2 cun lateral to the most outstanding vertebra on the neck.
Jiexi	ST 41	On the anterior aspect of both ankles, in the depression at the center of the front surface of the ankle joint, between the tendons of extensor hallucis longus and extensor digitorum longus.	In the depression of the junction of the dorsal foot and leg, between the two dorsal tendons.

Acupoint	Code	Location	Fast Localization
Jingming	BL 1	On both sides of the face, in the depression between the superomedial parts of the inner canthus of the eye and the medial wall of the orbit.	In sitting position, eyes closed, in the depression slightly above the inner corner of the eye on the finger palpation.
Jingbailao	EX-HN 15	On both sides of the neck, 2 cun straight superior to the seventh cervical spine, and 1 cun lateral to the middle line of the back.	Refer to the location.
Juliao	GB 29	Midpoint of the line connecting the anterior superior iliac spine and the prominence of the great trochanter on both sides of the body.	Midpoint between the anterior superior iliac spine and the great trochanter.
Kuan'gu	EX-LE 1	In front of both thighs, there are two points in each limb, and 1.5 cun later to Liangqiu point (ST 34).	Refer to the location.
Kunlun	BL 60	On the posterolateral aspect of both ankles, in the depression between the prominence of the later malleolus and the calcaneal tendon.	In sitting position, in the depression between the tip of the external malleolus and the Achilles tendon.

Acupoint	Code	Location	Fast Localization
Liangqiu	ST 34	On the anterolateral aspect of both thighs, between the vastus lateralis muscle and the lateral border of the rectus femoris tendon, 2 cun superior to the base of the patella.	In sitting position, extending forcefully and straightly the lower limbs, in the depression on the lateral superior border of the patella.
Mingmen	GV 4	In the lumbar region, in the depression inferior to the spinous process of the second lumbar vertebra, on the posterior midline.	In the depression on the posterior midline, right opposite to the umbilicus.
Naohui	TE 13	On the posterior aspect of both arms, posteroinferior to the border of the deltoid muscle, 3 cun inferior to the acromial angle.	On the line between Jianliao point (TE 14) and the tip of elbow, 4 cun below Jianliao point.
Neiguan	PC 6	On the anterior aspect of both forearms, between the tendons of the palmaris longus and the flexor carpi radialis, 2 cun proximal to the palmar wrist crease.	Wrist flexed slightly and fist made, 2 cun above the transverse crease of the wrist and between the two tendons.
Neixiyan	EX-LE 4	On both knees, and on the center of the depression of the patellar ligament.	Knee flexed, in the depression on the medial side of the patellar ligament.

Acupoint	Code	Location	Fast Localization
Qihaishu	BL 24	On both sides of the lumbar region, at the same level as the inferior border of the spinous process of the third lumbar vertebra, 1.5 cun lateral to the posterior midline.	1.5 cun lateral to the lower border of one more vertebra down from the vertebra at the same level of the umbilicus.
Qiuxu	GB 40	On the anterolateral aspect of both ankles, in the depression lateral to the extensor digitorum longus tendon, anterior and distal to the lateral malleolus.	In sitting or lying on the side, anterior inferior to the external malleolus, in the depression between the lateral side of the extensor digitorum longus tendon and heel joint.
Quchi	LI 11	On the lateral aspect of both elbows, at the midpoint of the line connecting Chize point (LU 5) with the lateral epicondyle of the humerus.	Arm flexed, at the end to the transverse cubital crease, close to the tip of elbow.
Quepen	ST 12	In the anterior region of the neck of both sides of body, in the greater supraclavicular fossa, 4 cun lateral to the anterior midline, in the depression superior to the clavicle.	Sitting straightly, the point is where the depression over the clavicle and on the mammillary line.

Acupoint	Code	Location	Fast Localization
Sanyinjiao	SP 6	On the tibial aspect of both legs, posterior to the medial border of the tibia, 3 cun superior to the prominence of the medial malleolus.	In a sitting or supine position, posterior to the medial border of the tibia, four fingers' breadth directly above the tip of the medial malleolus.
Shaohai	HT 3	On the anteromedial aspect of both elbows, just anterior to the medial epicondyle of the humerus, at the same level as the cubital crease.	Elbow flexed at 90°, in the depression on the medial end of the transverse cubital crease.
Shenmai	BL 62	On the lateral aspect of both feet, directly inferior to the prominence of the lateral malleolus, in the depression between the inferior border of the lateral malleolus and the calcaneus.	In sitting, in the depression directly below the external malleolus, feeling soreness and distention on pressure.
Shenmen	HT 7	On the anteromedial aspect of both wrists, radial to the flexor carpi ulnaris tendon, on the palmar wrist crease.	Loosely making a fist, hold the wrist with the hand and the thumb flexed. The point is in the depression where the nail touches the hand.

Acupoint	Code	Location	Fast Localization
Shousanli	LI 10	On the posterolateral aspect of both forearms, on the line connecting Yangxi point (LI 5) with Quchi point (LI 11), 2 cun inferior to the cubital crease.	Elbow flexed, 2 cun inferior to the end of the transverse cubital crease.
Taixi	KI 3	On the posteromedial aspect of both ankles, in the depression between the prominence of the medial malleolus and the calcaneal tendon.	In a sitting position, in the depression between the medial malleolus and the Achilles tendon.
Taiyang	EX-HN 5	At the temples on both sides of the head, between the tip of the brow and outer canthal, the depression that 1 cun behind and inferior to it.	In a sitting or supine position, in the depression lateral to the outer end of eyebrow.
Tianzhu	BL 10	In the posterior region of both sides of the neck, at the same level as the superior border of the spinous process of the second cervical vertebra, in the depression lateral to the trapezius muscle.	1.5 cun lateral to the posterior midline.

Acupoint	Code	Location	Fast Localization
Tianzong	SI 11	In the scapular region on both sides of the body, in the depression between the upper one-third and lower two-thirds of the line connecting the midpoint of the spine of the scapula with the inferior angle of the scapula.	Place the contralateral hand on the scapula from the neck and shoulder, the point is where the middle finger touches.
Tinggong	SI 19	On both sides of the face, in the depression between the anterior border of the center of the tragus and the posterior border of the condylar process of the mandible.	Open the mouth lightly, in the depression between the antilobium and the articulatio mandibularis.
Tinghui	GB 2	On both sides of the face, in the depression between the intertragic notch and the condylar process of the mandible.	In sitting, anterior and inferior to the tragus, in the depression when opening the mouth.
Waiguan	TE 5	On the posterior aspect of both forearms, 2 cun proximal to the dorsal wrist crease, midpoint of the interosseous space between the radius and the ulna.	Palm down, 2 cun directly above the midpoint of the transverse crease of the wrist, between two bones.

Acupoint	Code	Location	Fast Localization
Weizhong	BL 40	On the posterior aspect of both knees, at the midpoint of the popliteal crease.	On the back of knee, in the center of the popliteal crease.
Xiguan	LR 7	On the tibial aspect of both legs, inferior to the medial condyle of the tibia, 1 cun posterior to Yinlingquan point (SP 9).	1 cun posterior to Yinlingquan point (SP 9), in the depression.
Xiyangguan	GB 33	On the lateral aspect of two knees, in the depression between the biceps femoris tendon and the iliotibial band, posterior and proximal to the lateral epicondyle of the femur.	Knee flexed at 90°, in the depression superior to the bone on the lateral side of the knee.
Xuanzhong	GB 39	On the fibular aspect of both legs, anterior to the fibula, 3 cun proximal to the prominence of the lateral malleolus.	4 cun superior to the lateral malleolus, anterior to the fibula.
Xuehai	SP 10	On the anteromedial aspect of both thighs, on the bulge of the vastus medialis muscle, 2 cun superior to the medial end of the base of the patella.	When the patient's knee is flexed to an angle of 90°, cup your right palm to the left knee, with the other four fingers directed proximally, and the thumb forming an angle of 45°, the point is where the tip of your thumb rests.

Acupoint	Code	Location	Fast Localization
Yanglingquan	GB 34	On the fibular aspect of both legs, in the depression anterior and distal to the head of the fibula.	Bend knee flexed at 90°, on the lateral and inferior of the knee joint, in the depression anterior and inferior to the small head of the fibula.
Yangxi	LI 5	On the posterolateral aspect of the wrist, at the radial side of the dorsal wrist crease, distal to the radial styloid process, in the depression of the anatomical snuffbox.	Tilt the thumb, in the depression on the radial side of the wrist.
Yaoyangguan	GV 3	In the lumbar region, in the depression inferior to the spinous process of the fourth lumbar vertebra, on the posterior midline.	In a prone position, in the depression at the level of the spinous process of the uppermost ends of the hip joints.
Yaoshu	GV 2	In the sacral region, at the sacral hiatus, on the posterior midline.	In prone or lying on one side, on the posterior midline, at the level of two sacral angles (bilateral and superior to the coccyx).

Acupoint	Code	Location	Fast Localization
Yifeng	TE 17	In the anterior region of the neck, posterior to the two ear lobes, in the depression anterior to the inferior end of the mastoid process.	In the depression right posterior to the earlobe.
Yinlingquan	SP 9	On the tibial aspect of the leg, in the depression between the inferior border of the medial condyle of the tibia and the medial border of the tibia.	Push upward along the medial border on the medial side of the leg with the thumb, in the depression on the medial side of the tibia.
Yinmen	BL 37	On the posterior aspect of both thighs, between the biceps femoris and the semitendinosus muscle, 6 cun inferior to the gluteal fold.	Refer to the location.
Yintang	GV 29	In the forehead, at the depression of the middle of the two eyebrows' medial end.	The midpoint of the line between eyebrows.
Yongquan	KI 1	On the sole of both feet, in the deepest depression when the foot is in plantar flexion.	Foot flexed, in the depression on the anterior 1/3 on the sole.

Acupoint	Code	Location	Fast Localization
Yuzhen	BL 9	On both sides of the head, at the same level as the superior border of the external occipital protuberance, and 1.3 cun lateral to the posterior midline.	Refer to the location.
Zhishi	BL 52	In the lumbar region on both sides of the body, at the same level as the inferior border of the spinous process of the second lumbar vertebra, 3 cun lateral to the posterior midline.	4 cun lateral to the lower border of the vertebra at the level of the umbilicus.
Zusanli	ST 36	On the anterior aspect of both legs, on the line connecting Dubi point (ST 35) with Jiexi point (ST 41), 3 cun inferior to the Dubi point.	In a standing position, bend the body, match the web of the first and second interphalangeal fingers with the upper lateral border of the hand, place the rest fingers naturally downward, the point is where the tip of the middle finger touches.